v|a|d|e|m|e|c|u|m

D1378683

Handbook of Cardiac Pacing

Charles J. Love , M.D.
Ohio State University Medical Center
Columbus, Ohio

LANDES
BIOSCIENCE

AUSTIN, TEXAS
U.S.A.

VADEMECUM
Handbook of Cardiac Pacing
LANDES BIOSCIENCE
Austin

Please address all inquiries to the Publisher:
Landes Bioscience, 810 S. Church Street, Georgetown, Texas, U.S.A. 78626
Phone: 512/ 863 7762; FAX: 512/ 863 0081

ISBN: 1-57059-492-9

Library of Congress Cataloging-in-Publication Data
Love, Charles J.
    Handbook of cardiac pacing / Charles J. Love
        p. cm.
    Includes bibliographical references and index.
    ISBN 1-57059-492-9
    1. Cardiac pacing--Handbooks, manuals, etc. I. Title.
    [DNLM: 1. Pacemaker, Artificial. 2. Defibrillators, Implantable.
3. Cardiac Pacing, Artificial. WG 26L897h 1998]
RC684.P3L68 1998
617.4'120645--DC21
DNLM/DLC   98-26333
for Library of Congress   CIP

While the authors, editors, sponsor and publisher believe that drug selection and dosage and the specifications and usage of equipment and devices, as set forth in this book, are in accord with current recommendations and practice at the time of publication, they make no warranty, expressed or implied, with respect to material described in this book. In view of the ongoing research, equipment development, changes in governmental regulations and the rapid accumulation of information relating to the biomedical sciences, the reader is urged to carefully review and evaluate the information provided herein.

Dedication

With much thanks and love to my wife Jill and my children Aaron and Dara for their patience and understanding during the preparation of this manuscript. Daddy's back.

And

With my most sincere appreciation to Dr. Charles V. Meckstroth, a teacher and a friend.

And

With my respect, thanks and best wishes to the nurses and technologists at The Ohio State University Heart Center for their excellence and efforts towards the Arrhythmia Device Service. Janet, Kathy, Marg, Paul, Lee, John and Kelley —you're the best!

Contents

Foreword

This book is intended for the physician, nurse, student or technician that occasionally comes in contact with patients who have implanted heart rhythm control devices. It is meant as a reference and basic resource to provide quick explanations and answers to situations that are likely to be encountered relating to pacemakers and implantable cardioverter defibrillators. The terminology and language unique to the professionals who deal with these devices are presented and examples of basic and advanced pacemaker function are covered. Figures are used extensively to depict examples of normal and abnormal device function. Common malfunctions are described and an approach to the diagnosis and remedy of these problems is presented. The indications for the use of pacemakers and defibrillators are discussed as well as the contraindications. Surgical issues and patient concerns are covered. The rationale for follow up and the follow up procedures for these devices are explained.

Acknowledgments

A special thanks to Dennis Mathias for his assistance in the preparation of the graphics for this publication.

NASPE/BPEG Codes
for Permanent Pacing

In order to understand the "language" of pacing, it is necessary to comprehend the coding system that was developed originally by the International Conference on Heart Disease (commonly known as the ICHD) and subsequently modified by the NASPE/BPEG (North American Society of Pacing and Electrophysiology—British Pacing and Electrophysiology Group) alliance. The purpose of this coding system is to allow one to communicate the expected behavior of a pacing device to a health care worker or pacemaker technician quickly and accurately. Failure to understand these codes is common, especially as they relate to the more complex device functions. However, if one cannot communicate with a consultant quickly and accurately in this manner, improper evaluation of the pacemaker performance may result, with subsequent misdiagnosis and possibly improper treatment of the patient. A separate code has been developed for implantable cardioverter defibrillators and is discussed in chapter 11.

The NASPE/BPEG code (also known as the NBG code) consists of a five position system using a letter in each position to describe the programmed function of a pacing system (Table 1.1). For devices other than defibrillators and pacemakers with anti-tachycardia capability, only the first three or four positions are routinely used. The first position designates the chamber or chambers paced. It is useful to remember that the primary purpose of a pacemaker is to pace, and thus the first letter of the code represents this first function of the device. The letters used are V, A, D and O to designate Ventricle, Atrium, Dual chamber or Off.

The earliest pacemakers could only pace the heart. They had no ability to respond to a patient's own cardiac rhythm. It was soon found that pacing all of the time (asynchronously) not only wasted the limited battery power available, but could also result in the induction of tachyarrhythmias. This can occur when a pacemaker pulse is delivered during the vulnerable period of the cardiac cycle. This is analogous to an "R on T" premature ventricular contraction (PVC) that results in ventricular tachycardia. For these reasons it is beneficial to sense the native heart rhythm, and this is the secondary function of a modern pacemaker. The pacemaker pulse is delivered only when it is needed and withheld when an appropriate underlying rhythm is present. The letters used to designate the chambers being sensed are identical to those used for the chambers being paced; V, A, D and O, with the same meanings.

When an event is sensed by the pacing system a response to the sensed event may occur. The third letter of the NBG code describes how the pacemaker will respond to a sensed event. The letters used are I, T, D and O to designate Inhibited, Triggered (or Tracking), Dual response or Off (no response). The easiest response

1

Table 1.1. NASPE/BPEG (NBG) codes

1st position indicates the chamber paced:
V = ventricle
A = atrium
D = dual
O = no pacing

2nd position indicates the chamber sensed:
V = ventricle
A = atrium
D = dual
O = no sensing

3rd position indicates the response to a sensed event:
I = inhibited
T = triggered/tracking
D = dual
O = no response

4th position indicates programmability & rate response:
O = not programmable
P = simple programming (three functions or less)
M = multiprogrammable (more than three functions)
C = communicating (M + telemetry capabilities)
R = rate responsive

5th position indicates anti-tachyarrhythmia functions:
O = none
P = pacing
S = shock
D = dual (shock and pacing)

---

to understand is the inhibited response. If the pacemaker senses an event outside of a refractory period (see chapter 2), it inhibits the pacemaker and resets the device to start another timing cycle. A pacemaker programmed to the VVI mode would pace the ventricle, sense the ventricle, and if a sensed QRS occurred before the pacemaker stimulus was due, it would withhold the stimulus (i.e., be inhibited) and reset for another cycle. An AAI pacemaker is identical in all ways to a VVI pacemaker except for the fact that the pacing lead (wire) is placed in the atrium rather than the ventricle.

The triggered or tracking mode is often a source of confusion as it is not used in single chamber applications very often. Instead of inhibiting the output when the pacemaker senses an intrinsic event, a pace output is delivered when the sensed event occurs. In a VVT pacemaker the device will pace at the programmed rate unless a sensed QRS occurs. If a QRS is detected before the next pacing pulse is due to occur, the device will immediately deliver a pace output. The appearance will be a pacemaker pulse somewhere in the native QRS. AAT performs in the same fashion except it is triggered by P-wave sensing and paces the atrium.

In a DDD pacemaker (dual chamber pacing, dual chamber sensing, dual mode of response) the operation of the pacemaker is more complex as the atrial and ventricular channels must work together. Any sensed ventricular event will inhibit both atrial and ventricular outputs and reset the device for the next timing cycle. However, if an atrial event is sensed first, the atrial output is inhibited and a ventricular output will be triggered after a programmed interval. The ventricular output will be inhibited if a spontaneous ventricular event occurs before the end of this interval. This inhibited and triggered response is represented by the third "D" in the dual response designation of the code. Additional explanation of the codes with examples of timing diagrams are found in chapters 3 and 4.

The fourth position of the NBG code is used to designate the presence of certain programmable, communication or special features of the device. The designations are presumed to be hierarchical. If a device has a more advanced function it is presumed to have all of the lower functions as well (though this is not always true). The letter codes used in this position are O, P, M, C and R, nO-programmable features, Programmable for three or fewer parameters, Multiprogrammable (more than three parameters), Communicating with telemetry and Rate responsive (sensor-driven). It is common to use the fourth letter only when a rate modulation sensor is present. Thus, a VVIR pacemaker would have the capability to regulate the rate based on its own sensor, and a VVI pacemaker would only be able to pace at a fixed rate.

The fifth position is used to designate anti-tachycardia features. In a similar fashion to the fourth position it is used only when the feature is present and is otherwise omitted. The codes O, P, S and D are used. These describe nO anti-tachycardia features, anti-tachycardia Pacing, Shock capability, or Dual (pace and shock) capability, respectively.

Basic Concepts of Pacing

PACEMAKER COMPONENTS

BATTERY

The primary power source for permanent pacemakers has evolved from short-lived and unreliable chemistries to the long-lasting and durable ones that we use today. A common misconception is that when the battery is depleted that just this component is changed. In reality, the pacemaker is a welded, hermetically sealed can without any provision for replacement of individual components (Fig. 2.1). When the battery is depleted, or when any component of the pacemaker does not function properly, the entire device is replaced.

Mercury zinc batteries were used in early pacemakers. The pacemakers could not be hermetically sealed as these batteries produced gases over time that required venting. This resulted in fluid leakage into the pacemaker at times that caused electrical shorting and premature failure. Mercury zinc batteries have a fairly short useful life and have an abrupt drop in voltage as they become depleted. This would make predicting the pending failure of the batteries difficult. No devices of this type are currently in use.

Nuclear pacemakers use a very small amount of the highly toxic and radioactive element Plutonium to generate heat. The heat released on radioactive decay is converted into electricity by a thermocouple (Fig. 2.2). Though these devices had very long service lives (some were guaranteed for 72 years), they were large and created problems when traveling between states and countries due to the presence of their radioactive fuel. They must also be removed at the time of death and returned for proper disposal. Nuclear power sources became obsolete when the long lived lithium batteries were developed. Though nuclear powered pacemakers are no longer sold there are still a small number of nuclear devices that remain in use.

Rechargeable pacemakers use a nickel-cadmium battery that must be charged each week. The recharging is done using a method known as "inductive coupling". A coil is placed on the skin over the pacemaker which transfers energy to a coil within the device via electromagnetic waves. The pacemakers are large and have become obsolete with newer technology. There are still some rechargeable pacemakers in use though none are currently being sold.

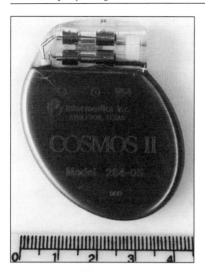

Fig. 2.1a. Photograph of a typical pacemaker. This device weighs only 24 grams (less than 1 ounce) and will last an average of 7 years.

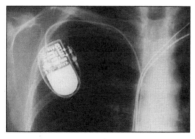

Fig. 2.1b. Radiograph of a typical pacemaker showing the battery and circuitry. The internal skeleton of a similar pacemaker shows the large battery (white), and the integrated circuitry.

Lithium iodine is currently the only power source being used in pacemakers today. This chemistry provides a long shelf life and high energy density (it can store a lot of power in a small space). Lithium cupric sulfide was used in some pacemakers manufactured by the Cordis Corporation due to its excellent energy density. However, due to the corrosive nature of this compound many abrupt pacemaker failures occurred when the battery chemicals ate through their containment. While still present in implanted devices, lithium cupric sulfide is no longer used. Lithium iodine has two other characteristics that make it an excellent power source. The self discharge rate is very low resulting in a long shelf life. It has a stable voltage through much of the useful life then tapers down in a gradual and predictable manner. This makes predicting the elective replacement time safe and easy.

Vanadium silver pentoxide is a newer compound that is used in implantable defibrillators. Though its energy density is not as high as lithium iodine, it has the ability to deliver a large amount of current very quickly. Currently this is the only power source used to charge the defibrillation capacitors. Though this type of

Fig. 2.2. Radiograph of a nuclear pacemaker. The plutonium is located in a central chamber. As the isotope decays it generates heat that is converted into electricity by a thermocouple. Note the marked difference in appearance from a "standard" pacemaker such as seen in Figure 2.1b.

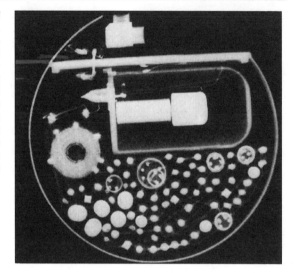

battery is good at rapid current delivery, it is not well suited to chronic low-level drains. Thus, some newer defibrillators are being made with two power sources: one for the shock circuit and one for the pacing and sensing circuit.

CIRCUITRY

Early devices were a mass of individual resistors, transistors and capacitors wired together or placed on printed circuit boards (Fig. 2.3a). New devices are now placed on "chips" and are controlled by microprocessors. They are essentially small computers with RAM and ROM (Fig. 2.3b). This has resulted in a marked decrease in size, weight, and power consumption. There has also been a tremendous increase in features, reliability, flexibility and longevity. The newer devices have tremendous data storage capabilities to track the function of the device as well as many different patient parameters. The latter includes total number of cardiac events, the rate of these events, whether these were paced or intrinsic, and the number of high-rate episodes (Fig. 2.4). The newest devices have the ability to store intracardiac electrograms and may function has "Holter" or event monitors with the ability to playback the paced or sensed events (Fig. 2.5). Current generation implantable defibrillators are capable of recording actual cardiogram strips during a symptomatic episode (Fig. 2.6). This same feature is now available in some pacemakers.

CONNECTOR BLOCK

The connector block (also referred to as the "header") is the means by which the pacemaker wire is connected to the pacemaker circuitry. As shown in Figure 2.7, there are many different sizes and styles of connector blocks. All types have in common a method for securing the wire to the pacemaker and a method

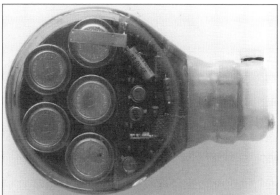

Fig. 2.3a. (above) Photograph of an older pacemaker showing the discrete components. This device was molded in epoxy and was transparent. The simple components and 5 mercury-zinc batteries are visible.

2

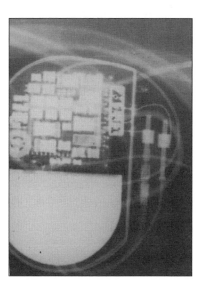

Fig. 2.3b. Radiograph of a newer pacemaker with integrated circuitry and microprocessor based design. This device has a single lithium battery for long service life and reliability. The case is made of titanium.

for making a secure electrical connection. If the wrong type of connector block is used the wire may not fit into it properly, the wire may loosen or the electrical connection may not be made. Any of these can result in a nonfunctioning pacing system. Most pacemakers use set screws to both attach the lead to the pacemaker and make the electrical connection at the same time. If a bipolar connection is to be made there may be one set screw for the anode and another for the cathode. As many as four set screws may be present in a dual chamber bipolar pacemaker. Another type of connector uses a set screw for the distal pin and a spring connector for the ring on the lead. The newest connectors do not use any screws. These have spring connectors for all of the electrical connections and a mechanism for gripping the lead body to hold it in place. The advantage to this system is that it

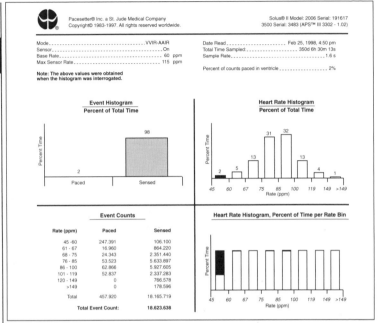

Fig. 2.4. Printout of pacemaker telemetry data shows the cardiac and paced events since the last evaluation. This pacemakeer is programmed to pace and sense the ventricle in a patient with chronic atrial fibrillation. Only 2% of the heartbeats that the patient actually had were caused by the pacemaker. The remaining 98% were intrinsic beats. This strip would be representative of a patient with atrial fibrillation and poor rate control suggesting that an increase in AV node blocking drugs (such as digitalis) or an AV node ablation would be appropriate.

makes the electrical connection "automatic," and does not rely on the physician to make a secure connection with a screw.

LEADS

Pacemaker leads are more than simple "wires." They are complex and highly engineered devices and consist of many components (Fig. 2.8). Figure 2.9 shows some of the many different types of leads that have evolved in an effort to reduce the size and increase the reliability of this critical pacing component. Each part of the lead is highly specialized and will be addressed individually below.

ELECTRODE

All pacemaker and ICD leads have one or more electrically active surfaces referred to as the electrode(s). The purpose the electrode is to deliver an electrical stimulus, detect intrinsic cardiac electrical activity, or both. The composition, shape and size of an electrode will vary quite widely from one model lead to another. A summary of the materials used is shown in Table 2.1. Many modern electrodes are

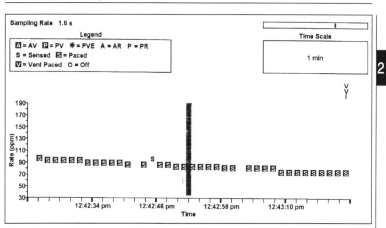

Fig. 2.5. Event record. This is "mini-Holter" that shows each cardiac event and the activity of the pacemaker at that instant. The patient's heart rate, the paced rate and the time are displayed. Patient symptoms may be correlated to the cardiac events that are recorded by the device.

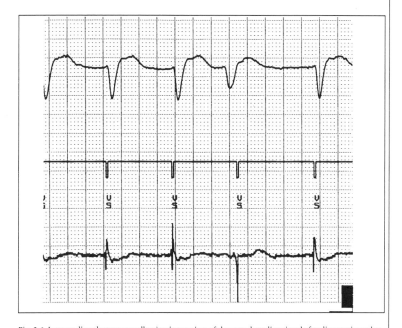

Fig. 2.6. Intracardiac electrogram allowing inspection of the actual cardiac signals for diagnostic evaluation. The top trace is the surface ECG, the bottom trace is the intracardiac electrogram. The middle trace shows the event marker. The markers annotate the events indicating whether the pacemaker is sensing or pacing during these events. In this case VS indicates a ventricular sensed event. Note the different appearance of the electrogram associated with the PVC.

Fig. 2.7. Connector block types. a. 2 set screws for each lead (total of 4 in this bipolar dual chamber device), one for the anode and cathode. Each screw must be tightened to hold the lead and provide a secure electrical connection.

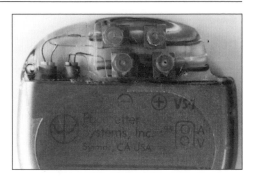

Fig. 2.7b. One set screw for each lead to hold the distal pin (cathode). The anode is connected electrically by a spring loaded band. A unipolar pacemaker would have only a single screw for each lead without the need for an anodal screw.

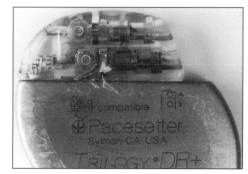

Fig. 2.7c. Nonscrew design uses spring loaded bands to contact both the cathode and the anode. A plastic component is presed in by hand that then grips the lead connector to prevent it from coming out of the connector block.

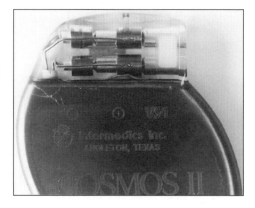

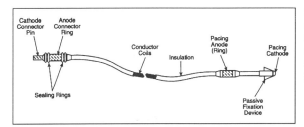

Fig. 2.8. Diagram of a typical bipolar pacing lead. The lead is a complex device with many different components.

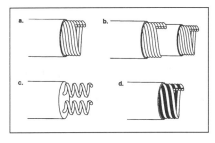

Fig. 2.9. Diagram of the four basic types of leads. a. Unipolar design with a single coil covered by an insulator. b. Coaxial bipolar design uses two concentric coils separated by a layer of insulation. c. Parallel bipolar design is similar to an electrical cord with the two conductors side by side. d. Coated coil bipolar design insulates each individual filament so they may be wound together giving the look and feel of a unipolar lead.

Table 2.1. Electrode types

elgiloy
polished platinum
micro porous platinum (platinized or "black" platinum)
macro porous platinum (mesh)
vitreous carbon
iridium oxide
platinum iridium
titanium nitride

---

designed to elute an anti-inflammatory drug such as dexamethasone sodium phosphate (Fig. 2.10). Eluting such a drug at the electrode surface has been shown to reduce the amount of acute inflammation and thus the amount of fibrosis at the electrode myocardial interface. Less fibrosis allows the electrode to remain in closer contact with the excitable myocardial cells. This provides a greater charge density and has the effect of reducing the amount of electrical current required to stimulate the muscle. The result is lower battery drain and increased longevity of the pacemaker by allowing the pacemaker output to be reduced.

INSULATION

One of the most important components of any lead system is the insulation. The insulation prevents electrical shorting between the conductor coils within the lead, prevents stimulation of tissues other than the heart and allows smooth passage of the lead into the vein. Failure of the insulation may result in a number of different problems, the most important of which is failure to pace. Several hundred thousand pacing leads are on alert or recall due to a high rate of insulation

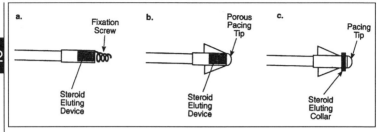

Fig. 2.10. Diagram of steroid eluting lead designs. a. Active fixation tip with steroid behind the screw. b. Passive fixation tip with steroid behind the tip. c. Passive fixation tip with steroid around the tip.

Table 2.2. Insulation types

silicone / silastic
80A polyurethane
55D polyurethane
other polyurethanes
Teflon "coated coil" technology

---

failure. Most of these are coaxial bipolar leads with 80A Pellathane™ polyurethane as the insulator between the two coils. This particular type of polyurethane is subject to metal ion oxidation (MIO) and environmental stress cracking (ESC). MIO is a reaction catalyzed by the metals of the conductor coil. It results in a breakdown of the polyurethane such that it will fail to be capable of insulating. This was found to be most prevalent in leads that utilized silver in the conductor coil. ESC may be severe and result in cracks in the insulation and electrical shorting. It is critical that patients with these lower reliability leads be identified and followed appropriately. In some cases prophylactic replacement may be indicated. The newest methodology to insulate leads is known as "coated coil" insulation. This technology bonds an insulating coat to each individual filament of the wire. The whole wire is then covered with a more standard insulator. Even if this outer coating is breached, the individual filaments remain electrically isolated. The types of insulation commonly in use are listed in Table 2.2.

CONDUCTOR COIL

The metal portion of the wire that carries electrical signals to and from the pacemaker and the electrode is the conductor coil. Most coils are made of multifilar (several strands) components, as shown in Figure 2.11. This provides strength and flexibility as compared with a solid wire (for example a coat hanger is a solid wire while a lamp cord is multifilar). As the conductor coils are constantly flexed in and around the heart as well as under the clavicle or rib margin, fractures may occur. This may lead to a complete or intermittent loss of pacing. Multiple conductor coils may be present in a lead. The more coils that are present, the more complex the lead construction and therefore the less reliable the lead.

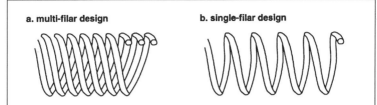

Fig. 2.11a. Multifilar design is made up of several thin filiments of wire twisted together providing both strength and flexibility. b. Single filar design is similar to a coat hanger. It can be fractured easily by repeated bending and flexing.

Table 2.3. Fixation mechanisms

none ("kerplunk" leads)
tines
fins
talons
cones
flanges
fixed extended helix
retractable helix
specialized shape (e.g., preformed "J")

FIXATION

Once the lead is placed, there is usually some type of fixation mechanism present to prevent the lead from dislodging (Table 2.3, Fig. 2.12). Early lead designs did not have a fixation mechanism and were often referred to as "kerplunk" leads since they were heavy and stiff thus dropping into position. Newer leads have either a passive mechanism that entangles the lead into the trabeculations or a helix that can be screwed into the myocardium. The helix may be extendible and retractable, or may be fixed to the end of the lead.

CONNECTOR

The portion of the lead that connects it to the pacemaker is known as the connector. There are many types of connectors (Table 2.4, Fig. 2.13), and thus the opportunity for confusion and mismatches exists. It is imperative that the implanting physician understand the differences and issues involving the connectors. Currently, all manufacturers have agreed upon the International Standard-1 (IS-1). Prior to the IS-1 designation, a voluntary standard had been established (VS-1), however these two designations are virtually identical. This is finally eliminating the confusion generated by decades of proprietary designs. Thus, an IS-1 lead from one manufacturer should be compatible with an IS-1 connector block of another manufacturer.

Fig. 2.12. Fixation types. a. Plain leads had no fixation device and were held in place by their weight and stiffness. b. Tines were added to act as a "grappling hook" to reduce dislodgment. c. Fins are a variation on tines. These may be less likely to become entanled in the valve. d. Fixed helix active fixation leads screw in to the myocardium by rotating the entire lead. The helix is always out. Some manufacturers coat the helix with an inert and rapidly dissolving substance (such as a sugar) to protect the helix during insertion. e. Extendable helix leads have a mechanism to extend and retract the screw. f. Preformed "J" lead for simplified atrial placement.

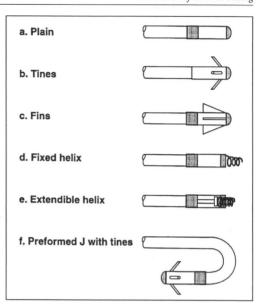

a. Plain

b. Tines

c. Fins

d. Fixed helix

e. Extendible helix

f. Preformed J with tines

Table 2.4. Connector types

6 mm unipolar
6 mm inline bipolar
5 mm unipolar
5 mm inline bipolar
5 mm bifurcated bipolar
3.2 mm unipolar
3.2 mm inline bipolar
Medtronic/CPI type (no seals, long pin)
Cordis type (seals, long pin)
VS-1 / IS-1 (seals, short pin)

Fig. 2.13. Connector types: a. 5 mm unipolar; b. 5 mm bifurcated bipolar; c. 3.2 mm "low profile" in-line bipolar uses a long cathode pin but no sealing rings; d. 3.2 mm "Cordis Type" in-line bipolar uses a long cathode pin and sealing rings; e. 3.2 mm IS-1 in-line bipolar uses a short cathode pin and sealing rings.

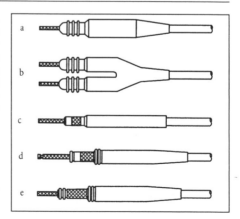

UNIPOLAR AND BIPOLAR PACING SYSTEMS

All electrical circuits must have a cathode (negative pole) and an anode (positive pole). In general, there are two types of pacing systems with reference to where the anode is located. One type of system, as shown in Figure 2.14a, uses the metal can of the pacemaker as the anode (+), and the wire as the cathode (−). This is referred to as a UNIPOLAR system, as the lead has only one electrical pole. Figure 2.14b shows the other type of system where both the anode (+) and the cathode (−) are on the pacing lead. This is referred to as a BIPOLAR system. In all pacing systems the distal pole that is in contact with the heart muscle is negative.

Unipolar systems have the advantage of a simpler (and possibly more reliable) single coil lead construction. It is also much easier to see the pace artifact with a unipolar system as the distance between the two poles is long and the electrical path is closer to the skin surface. In some cases sensing and capture thresholds may be better than in bipolar systems, though the lead impedance (pacing resistance) may be lower resulting in higher current drain from the battery.

Bipolar systems have several characteristics that have made this polarity choice increasingly popular. This has been especially true as dual chamber pacing has become more prevalent. Because the distance between the electrodes is small (short antenna) and since the electrodes are both located deep within the body, these devices are much more resistant to electrical interference caused by skeletal muscle activity or electromagnetic interference (EMI) relative to unipolar systems. Also, at higher output settings one may have stimulation of the pocket around the pacemaker in a unipolar system. This is virtually unknown in normally functioning bipolar systems. The one complaint that is often heard about the bipolar pacing polarity is that the pace artifact is very small on the electrocardiogram. This makes determination of function and malfunction more difficult. For this reason it is not uncommon to see a pacemaker programmed to pace in the unipolar polarity and to sense in the bipolar polarity.

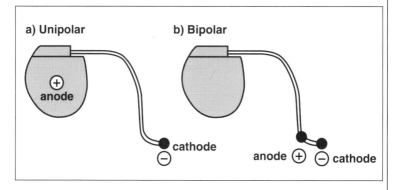

Fig. 2.14a. Unipolar pacing system. The lead tip is the cathode and the pacemaker case is the anode. b. Bipolar pacing system. The lead tip is the cathode and the anode is a ring slightly behind the cathode. The pacemaker case is not part of the pacing circuit.

BASIC CONCEPTS AND TERMS

PACING THRESHOLD

This is the minimum amount of energy required to consistently cause depolarization and therefore contraction of the heart. Pacing threshold is measured in terms of both amplitude (the strength of the impulse) and the duration of time for which it is applied to the myocardium (Fig. 2.15). The amplitude is most commonly programmed in volts (V), however some devices still use milliamps (mA) as the adjustable parameter. The duration is always measured in milliseconds (msec). A pacemaker that is adjustable for voltage output will always deliver the programmed voltage. The current delivered (mA) will vary with the resistance (in pacing this is referred to as impedance) of the lead system in accordance with Ohm's Law:

Volts = Current x Resistance (or) V=IR

The latter are thus called "constant voltage" devices. Other devices (such as many temporary pacemakers) are adjustable for their current in mA. These are called "constant current", as the current delivered remains fixed and the voltage will depend on the impedance of the lead system.

The strength-duration curve is a property of a given lead in a specific patient at a single point in time. An example of one of these curves is shown in Figure 2.16. The shorter the pulse width (duration) of an impulse, the higher the voltage or current (strength) needed to cause depolarization of the heart. The relation of these two parameters changes as the lead matures from acute at implant to chronic, moving the curve up and to the right. There may be additional changes during significant metabolic or physiologic abnormalities at the lead to myocardial interface. Some medications may also affect the threshold for capture (Table 2.5).

SENSING

Sensing is the ability of the device to detect an intrinsic beat of the heart. This purameter is measured in millivolts (mV). The larger the R-wave or P-wave in mV, the easier it is for the device to sense the event as well as to discriminate it from spurious electrical signals. Setting the sensitivity of a pacemaker is often confusing. When programming this value it must be understood that this is the

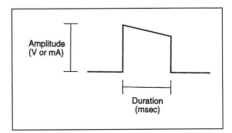

Fig. 2.15. Truncated exponential waveform. This magnified view of a pacing impulse has both a strength (or amplitude) measured in Volts or milliamps, as well as a duration measured in milliseconds. This type of waveform is used in both pacing and defibrillation applications.

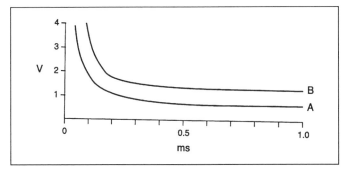

Fig. 2.16. Strength-Duration Curve. Curve A represents a series of measurements taken at the time of implant. Curve B represents the same lead after it has been implanted for 2 weeks. As the lead matures, the threshold rises causing the curve to move up and to the right. Each curve represents the threshold value. Settings that are on or above the line will cause a cardiac contraction while those below the line will not. Note that at some point, though one may continue to increase the pulse width, no further reduction in voltage threshold occurs.

Table 2.5. Medication effects on capture

Medication effects on capture
Drugs that increase capture threshold:
    Amiodarone
    Bretylium
    Encainide
    Flecainide
    Moricizine
    Propafenone
    Sotalol
Drugs that possibly increase capture threshold
    Beta blockers
    Lidocaine
    Procainamide
    Quinidine
Drugs that decrease capture threshold
    Atropine
    Epinepherine
    Isoproterenol
    Corticosteroids

smallest amplitude signal that will be sensed. There is an inverse relation between the setting and the sensitivity. The higher values are the less sensitive settings. Thus, a setting of 8mV requires *at least* an 8mV electrical signal for the pacemaker to see it. A 2mV setting will allow any signal above 2mV to be sensed (Fig. 2.17).

One question that frequently arises is, when does sensing of an intrinsic QRS actually occur? The answer to this is that it varies greatly from one patient to the next, and also within the same patient depending on where the electrical depolarization originates. The pacing lead does not see a QRS or P-wave as we see it on

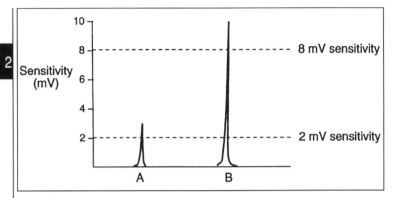

Fig. 2.17. Concept of sensitivity. Electrogram A is 3 millivolts in size and electrogram B is 10 millivolts in size. At a sensitivity setting of 2 mV both electrical signals have sufficient amplitude to be sensed. At a setting of 8 mV, only the larger signal will be sensed. Note that the higher the numerical value of the setting, the lower the sensitivity of the device to electrical signals.

the surface ECG. It sees an intracardiac electrogram (Fig. 2.18) that is more like a "spike." This spike occurs when the electrical depolarization within the heart passes by the electrode. For example, a PVC that comes from a focus in the right ventricle will be sensed very early in the QRS complex by a lead located in the right ventricle. Conversely, a PVC from the left ventricle will be sensed much later by that same electrode. Thus, when working with calipers on a surface ECG strip to determine proper device function, one may not be able to determine the exact point of sensing in many cases. One tool to assist in finding this point is the pacemaker programmer. The pacemaker can telemeter the exact point of sensing and mark the surface QRS for reference (Fig. 2.19).

SLEW RATE
Measurement of the intrinsic electrical signal for sensing is not simple as the pacemaker does not use all of the signal that is present. This "raw" electrical signal is filtered to eliminate a majority of noncardiac signals. Because the filtering allows only signals that have certain frequency content through to the sensing circuit, the final "filtered" signal may be substantially less than the original (Fig 2.20). One way of measuring the quality of the sensed signal is by looking at the "slew rate." This refers to the slope of the intrinsic signal and is measured in volts/second. High slew rates (> 1.0 V/sec in the ventricle and > 0.5 V/sec in the atrium) are desirable at implant for consistent sensing.

IMPEDANCE
In pacing, resistance (R) is referred to as impedance. The impedance of the lead to flow of current is caused by a combination of resistance in the lead, resistance through the patient tissues, and the "polarization" that takes place when

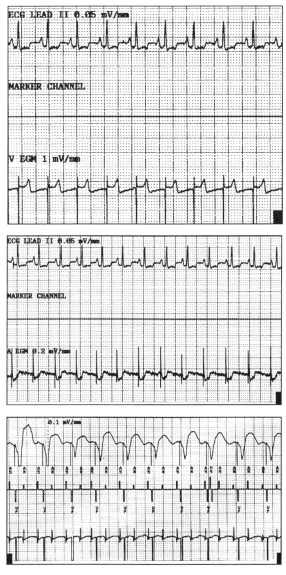

Fig. 2.18. Comparison of surface cardiogram and intracardiac electrogram recordings. Tracing A shows sinus rhythm with the normal QRS on top and the intracardiac ventricular electrogram on the bottom. Tracing B shows the intracardiac atrial electrogram on the bottom. These tracings were recorded at 12.5 mm/sec speed. Tracing C shows a paced rhythm with the intracardiac atrial electrogram on the bottom. This tracing reveals that the atrium is in a slow flutter rhythm. This trace was recorded at 25 mm/sec speed.

2

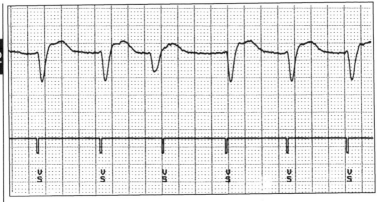

Fig. 2.19. Surface cardiogram recording (top) of a patient left bundle branch block and a PVC with a right bundle branch block morphology (3rd beat from the left). Annotation (bottom) is provided by the pacemaker showing the point at which the pacemaker actually senses the QRS (VS = ventricular sensed event). As the depolarization begins in the left ventricle when there is a right bundle branch block, the right ventricle depolarizes last. Note that the sense marker of the PVC occurs near the end of the surface QRS complex. Since the pacing lead is in the right ventricle, the pacemaker senses the beat late in the QRS.

Fig. 2.20a. Raw and filtered electrograms as telemetered from a pacemaker. The top trace is the filtered signal and is the one that is actually used by the pacemaker for sensing. Filtering of the raw signal (bottom trace) is necessary to prevent sensing of T-waves, far filed QRS signals and myopotentials (see text).

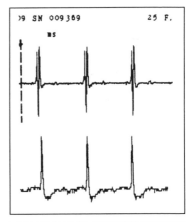

Fig. 2.20b. Comparison of a signal with a good slew rate (complex on the left) and one with a poor slew rate. The signal with the poor slew rate is broad and contains less high frequencey energy. Even though it is the same height as the good complex, it will not be sensed well as it will be stongly attenuated by the filtering of the pacemaker.

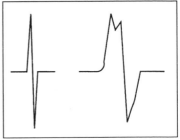

voltage and current are delivered into living tissue. An abrupt change in impedance may indicate a problem with the lead system. Very high resistance can indicate a conductor fracture or poor connection to the pacemaker. A very low resistance can indicate an insulation failure (Note: remember with Ohm's Law that V=IR or R=V/I). It is important to note that "normal" lead impedance may vary greatly from one lead to the next (250 to 2000 ohms) depending on the particular lead model and the method used to measure the impedance. Thus, a single impedance value may be of little use without previous values for comparison.

ACUTE IMPLANT VALUES

It is recommended at implant that capture thresholds be less than 1.0 V @ .5 msec. The standard method to obtain the threshold is by increasing the output until capture is obtained. However, if the patient has no underlying rhythm this must be done by decreasing the output until capture is lost then quickly increasing it. If a temporary pacemaker is present then the standard method may be used. The sensing threshold should be at least twice the nominal (standard) value for the device implanted, or an R-wave (≥5.0 mV and a P-wave ≥2.0 mV. These values may be difficult to achieve in some patients due to the presence of severe myocardial disease or endocardial fibrosis.

POSTIMPLANT VALUES

Capture thresholds typically rise for the first several weeks for most pacing leads, and then decline progressively towards their chronic values (Fig. 2.21). Some leads are designed with a method of delivering a small dose of steroid from the electrode tip to reduce the inflammatory response at the myocardial interface. These steroid eluting leads tend not to have a significant threshold rise during the acute period. The chronic phase for most leads is reached at 4 to 6 weeks postimplant. Due to the possibility of a threshold rise, the programmed output must provide a large safety margin during the acute phase to prevent a loss of capture. The output may then be adjusted to a lower value during the postoperative

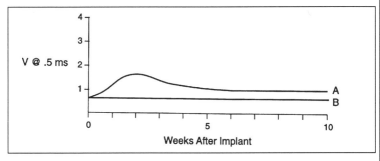

Fig. 2.21. Capture threshold versus time plot. Curve A is typical of older leads showing a threshold rise and fall during the four to six week period after implant. Curve B is typical of a modern technology lead, such as one with steroid elution. Little or no threshold rise is present due to the anti-inflammatory action of the steroid.

clinic visit one month later to prolong the life of the battery. Even if a steroid lead is used it may be wise to use the higher output initially should dislodgment of the lead occur.

PACING INTERVALS

Although we tend to think of cardiac cycles in terms of "beats per minute" (bpm), the pacemaker generally works in units of milliseconds (msec). Some parameters such as the lower and upper rate are programmed in bpm, while most other parameters are set in msec. When evaluating the device function, one must work with msec to determine if an event is occurring at the proper time.

An easy way to convert from bpm to msec or the reverse is the "Rule of 60,000." There are 1000 msec in a second, thus there are 60,000 msec in a minute. Dividing 60,000 by the bpm will result in the msec. Conversely, dividing 60,000 by the msec will yield the bpm (Fig. 2.22).

PROGRAMMABILITY

When permanent pacemakers were first implanted in 1958 there was no provision to change any parameter. The device was built to pace at one rate and output at the factory and remained at these values for the life of the device. As the patient presents a dynamic physiologic system with changing needs, the ability to change certain values such as the pacing rate and output amplitude became an obvious next step in pacemaker evolution. The first method of changing a device setting required placing a triangular needle through the skin into a receptacle on the pacemaker to make the adjustment. Shortly thereafter, using magnetic fields and then radiofrequency transmissions became the method. Programmability provides flexibility to decrease battery drain, correct abnormal device behavior and adapt the device to patient's specific and changing needs.

Basic programmable features are listed in Table 2.6. These are features that are present on virtually all pacemakers sold in nonthird world countries. Additional parameters are also listed in this table and may be available depending on the make and model of the device implanted. The cost of the pacemaker is usually proportional to the degree of programmability and the complexity of the built-in

---

60,000 Rule: 60,000 msec in a minute
60,000/Heart Rate = Interval in milliseconds
60,000/Interval in milliseconds = Heart rate

Examples:
Heart rate = 70 bpm
60,000/70 = 857 msec cycle length

Cycle Length = 857 msce
60,000/857 = 70 bpm

Fig. 2.22. Rate vs Interval: The Rule of 60,000.

Table 2.6. Programmable features

Basic
Mode
Rate
Output (V or mA)
Pulse Width
Sensitivity
Refractory Period

Advanced
Additional rate settings
Hysteresis rate (or interval)
Sleep rate
Sensor-driven Rate Settings
Maximum rate
Intermediate rate
Threshold
Slope or Rate Response Factor
Reaction Time (Acceleration time)
Recovery Time (Deceleration time)
Other Sensor Specific Settings
Dual Chamber Parameters
Upper Rate Limit (maximum tracking rate)
A-V Delay
Adaptive
Differential
Positive Hysteresis
Negative Hysteresis
Postventricular Atrial Refractory Period (PVARP)
PMT Options
PVARP Extension on PVC (also "PEPVARP")
DVI on PVC (previously "DDX")
Blanking Period
Rate Smoothing
Fallback Rate
Fallback Slope
Miscellaneous
Lead Polarity
Automatic Mode Swtiching
Histogram Settings
Other Refractory Periods
Other Features

---

diagnostic capability. The function of these programmable features will be explained in later chapters.

MAGNET RESPONSE

All pacemakers have an internal switch that can be activated by the application of an appropriate magnet directly over the device. The response to magnet application varies for each pacemaker model and with the programmed mode. There is a great misconception by many people that placing a magnet over the pacemaker will turn it off. I once had a physician tell me "I have six magnets stacked on top of this guy's pacemaker and it is still pacing!" The fact is that virtually all pacemakers will pace asynchronously (sensing is disabled) with the application of a magnet (Fig. 2.23). The rate of pacing may change during the magnet application. It may be higher, lower or equal to the programmed rate depending on the device. In addition, be aware that in dual chamber devices the AV-interval and/or the mode of pacing may change (i.e., DDD to VOO instead of the expected DOO). The magnet rate is one method used to determine the status of the battery. Application of the magnet elicits pacing at a specific rate as defined by the model (and sometimes serial number). A change in this "magnet rate" according to the specification by the manufacturer will indicate an intensified follow-up period, recommended replacement time (RRT) or end of device life (EOL). Use of the magnet rate allows some determination of device status by simple transtelephonic transmission of a cardiac rhythm strip. Some devices allow the magnet response to be programmed "On" or "Off." If the response is programmed off, there will be NO response to magnet application.

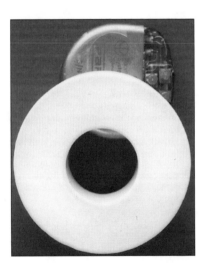

Fig. 2.23a. A ring magnet is shown in proper position placed over a pacemaker to close the magnetic reed switch within the pacemaker.

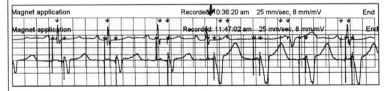

Fig. 2.23b. Strip showing magnet response of a pacemaker. The device paces in an asynchronous manner (no sensing of the underlying QRS or P waves). In this example, due to 100% AV pacing, this is ot readily seen. The clue to the change in this device is the shortening of the AVI which changes from 200 ms to 120 ms. The response of each manufacturer and model to the magnet may be unique.

Basic Single Chamber Pacing

3

BASIC PACING: SINGLE CHAMBER MODES

In order to understand the basic timing of a pacemaker one must understand the terminology commonly used to describe the events that occur. All single chamber pacemakers have three basic timed events:

Automatic Interval: The period of time between two sequential paced beats uninterrupted by a sensed beat (Fig. 3.1). It is also referred to as the base pacing interval and may be converted to bpm and expressed as the base pacing rate.

Escape Interval: The period of time after a sensed event until the next paced event (Fig. 3.2). The escape interval is usually the same as the automatic interval. It may be different if a feature called "hysteresis" is enabled (see below).

Refractory Period: This is a period of time after a paced or sensed event during which the pacemaker sensing is disabled (i.e., the pacemaker is refractory to external stimuli). An event occurring during a refractory period will not be sensed. This is done to prevent the pacemaker from sensing of the evoked QRS and T-wave for ventricular pacemakers. In atrial pacemakers the refractory period prevents sensing of the far-field R-wave or T-wave. Long refractory periods may prevent sensing of an early intrinsic beat such as a PAC or PVC (Fig. 3.3).

The most common single chamber mode is the VVI mode. As described by the NBG code the <u>V</u>entricle is paced and the <u>V</u>entricle is sensed. When an intrinsic beat is sensed the device will <u>I</u>nhibit the output and reset the timing cycle. The device function in the VVI mode is shown in Figure 3.4.

A much less common mode of pacing the ventricle is VVT. In this mode the <u>V</u>entricle is paced and the <u>V</u>entricle is sensed. If a sensed event occurs the pacemaker will <u>T</u>rigger a paced output immediately. If there is no intrinsic rhythm the pacemaker will pace at the programmed rate and be indistinguishable from a device programmed to the VVI mode (Fig. 3.5). Remember that in VVT any sensed event, either intrinsic QRS or an external electrical event that is strong enough to be sensed, will cause the pacemaker to deliver an output at that instant (i.e., it will be triggered). This mode is primarily used for diagnostic reasons. It may also be used to overdrive pace a tachycardia. This is done by placing two surface electrocardiogram electrodes near the pacemaker. These are attached by a wire to a temporary pacemaker or other stimulation source. Each time the pacemaker senses one of these external stimuli it will immediately pace the heart. This technique can be used to overdrive pace monomorphic ventricular tachycardia or to perform

Handbook of Cardiac Pacing, by Charles J. Love. © 1998 Landes Bioscience

Fig. 3.1. Automatic interval. This is the period
of time from one paced beat to the next paced
beat. In this example, the automatic interval is
1000 msec (or 60 beats per minute).

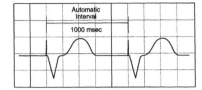

Fig. 3.2. Escape interval. This is the period of
time from when an intrinsic beat is sensed until
a paced beat will occur. In this example the escape interval is 1000 msec (or 60 beats per
minute).

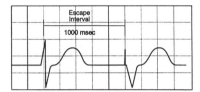

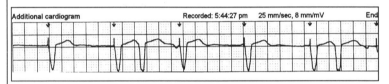

Fig. 3.3. Refractory period. The pacemaker will not respond to an intrinsic beat that occurs during the
pacemaker refractory period. In this example the pacemaker is set to VVI at 55 bpm. The refractory period has been programmed to 475 msec. QRS #3 and #7 are PVCs that fall within the refractory period of
the preceding paced beats. Since the pacemaker sensing is refractory during the PVC, the PVC is not
sensed. This is a programming problem, not a malfunction of the pacemaker.

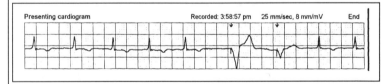

Fig. 3.4. VVI pacing @ 75 bpm. The ventricle is paced and sensed. An intrinsic beat inhibits the paced
output.

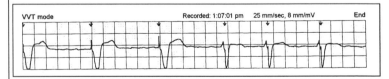

Fig. 3.5. VVT pacing @ 50 bpm. The ventricle is paced and sensed. The pacemaker will pace at the lower
rate limit. However, an intrinsic beat triggers an immediate output from the pacemaker.

programmed ventricular stimulation as with electrophysiologic studies. The upper rate of pacing is limited by the refractory period of the pacemaker and the runaway protection feature of the circuitry (see chapter 11). Some devices allow the runaway protection to be disabled temporarily during therapeutic VVT pacing.

VOO represents the "original pacing mode." In this mode of operation, the <u>V</u>entricle is paced, there is no sensing and thus there is no response to a sensed event (Fig. 3.6). VOO is a common mode of response in a ventricular pacemaker when a magnet is placed over a device programmed VVI or VVT. This causes pacing to occur asynchronously at a specific rate relative to the pacemaker model regardless of the underlying rhythm. The earliest pacemakers functioned in this fashion all of the time. The major drawback to a device functioning in the VOO mode continuously is that there may be competition with the patient's own rhythm. This may waste considerable battery power if the patient has a good intrinsic heart rate most of the time. It may also result in the induction of arrhythmias by pacing during the vulnerable period. This would be similar to the "R on T" phenomenon that results in ventricular tachycardia for some patients. VOO is only rarely programmed as a continuous mode of operation. It may be used for a patient that is pacemaker dependent (has no significant intrinsic rate of their own above 40 beats per minute) when oversensing or inappropriate inhibition of the device is suspected.

The atrial single chamber modes operate identically to the ventricular modes. The same pacemaker is used for atrial or ventricular applications, the difference being in which chamber the lead is placed.

The AAI mode (Fig. 3.7) operates just as the VVI mode, except that it paces the <u>A</u>trium, senses the <u>A</u>trium, and is <u>I</u>nhibited by P-waves instead of R-waves.

The AAT mode, as with the VVT mode, is used only for diagnostic or therapeutic reasons. A device programmed to AAT will pace the <u>A</u>trium, sense the <u>A</u>trium, and will <u>T</u>rigger a paced output when any electrical event is sensed on the

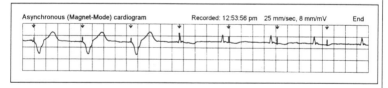

Fig. 3.6. VOO pacing. The ventricle is paced and there is no sensing of intrinsic beats. This is seen most often during the application of a magnet.

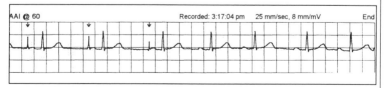

Fig. 3.7. AAI Pacing @ 60 bpm. The atrium is paced and sensed. An intrinsic beat inhibits the paced output.

atrial lead. If the intrinsic heart rate is slower than the programmed rate of the pacemaker, the appearance will be steady atrial pacing at the programmed rate (Fig.3.8).

Finally, the AOO mode paces asynchronously (without regard to the underlying rhythm) and is shown in Figure 3.9. It paces the <u>A</u>trium, but there is no sensing or response to sensed events. As with VOO pacing, this mode is seen with magnet application. It may also result in competition with the native rhythm and thus cause atrial arrhythmias and unnecessary battery wear.

ADDITIONAL CONCEPTS

HYSTERESIS

Hysteresis allows the pacemaker to refrain from pacing until a special lower rate known as the hysteresis rate is reached. When the hysteresis rate is reached the device then paces at the higher automatic rate until it is inhibited by a sensed event. Once inhibited, the hysteresis rate is "reset" and the device will not pace until the lower hysteresis rate is again reached (Fig. 3.10). It is in this situation that the escape interval is longer than the automatic interval. Some people prefer to think of the pacemaker as adding a hysteresis interval to the automatic interval rather than there being two different rates. Hysteresis is useful in patients with ventricular pacemakers and sinus rhythm who have infrequent pacing needs. It may also be useful when a ventricular pacemaker causes symptoms in a patient during pacing (see section on pacemaker syndrome in chapter 11).

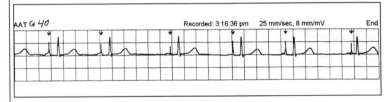

Fig. 3.8. AAT Pacing. The atrium is paced and sensed. An intrinsic beat triggers an immediate output from the pacemaker. Note the irregularity of the pacing interval. This is due to the patient's sinus arrhythmia and PACs.

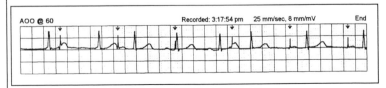

Fig. 3.9. AOO pacing. The atrium is paced and there is no sensing of intrinsic beats. This is seen most often during the application of a magnet.

FUSION AND PSEUDOFUSION

Fusion occurs when an intrinsic heart beat and a paced impulse occur at the same or nearly the same time (Fig. 3.11). The resultant QRS will resemble a standard paced beat if intrinsic conduction occurred late. Conversely, the QRS will more closely resemble the patient's own QRS if intrinsic conduction occurs early. If the paced impulse has no effect on the intrinsic QRS or T-wave, it is referred to as "pseudofusion" (Fig. 3.12) as no true fusion actually occurs. The presence of fusion and pseudofusion is frequently misinterpreted as a malfunction. This is usually not the case. As noted in chapter two, sensing of an intrinsic beat may not

3

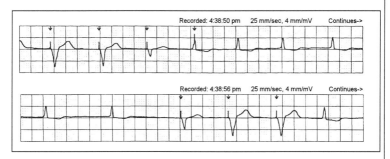

Fig. 3.10. Hysteresis. This is the one time when the escape interval is longer than the automatic interval. In this example the automatic rate is set to 70 bpm and the hysteresis rate is set to 50 bpm. The device paces at 70 bpm until inhibited by a sensed beat (5th beat on the top strip). It does not begin to pace again until the patient's intrinsic rate falls to 50 bpm (3rd beat on the bottom strip). The pace maker then paces at 70 bpm until another intrinsic beat is sensed (last beat on the bottom strip), at which time the hysteresis rate of 50 bpm is restored.

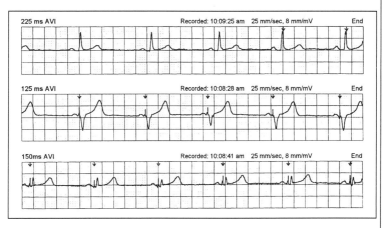

Fig. 3.11. Fusion. These three strips wre recorded from the same patient. The top strip shows the intrinsic QRS without any pacing. The second strip shows a strip with a paced QRS. The bottom strip shows a fused QRS that is intermediate between the paced and nonpaced complexes.

occur until late in the complex. Thus, even though the intrinsic QRS has started, the pacemaker may deliver an output as the depolarization has not reached the electrode by the time the paced output is due to occur. Only when the pulse clearly appears in the ST segment or T-wave can one be certain that failure to sense is present.

LATENCY

Latency is an uncommon phenomenon usually associated with metabolic derangement. It is when the pacemaker output spike occurs and captures; however there is a period (latent period) of isoelectric baseline prior to the QRS or P-wave following the spike (Fig. 3.13). Latency is also seen at other times such as in patients with severe intramyocardial conduction delays. As with fusion, this does not suggest a problem with the pacing system.

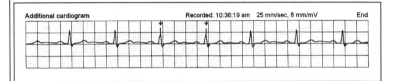

Fig. 3.12. Pseudofusion. The arrows show 2 paced outputs that occurred after the intrinsic complex is formed. The pace output does not affect the depolarization or repolarization of the heart (if it does then it is a fusion beat or a paced beat). This is often seen in normally functioning pacemakers, though in some situations it may also represent a malfunction.

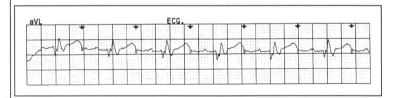

Fig. 13.13. Latency. This strip is recorded from a patient being paced in the atrium. Note the pause between the pace artifact (arrows) and the evoked P-wave. This patient had a significant metabolic abnormality at the time this tracing was recorded.

Dual Chamber Pacing

DUAL CHAMBER CONCEPTS AND MODES

Dual chamber devices are significantly more complex than their single chamber cousins. There are several additional timing intervals that are added and there are interactions between the timers. There are also two different methods for determining the basic timing of the device. Ventricular based timing has historically been the most common. However, with the newer sensor-driven dual chamber devices atrial based timing is becoming more common.

AV-Interval (AVI)

The AV-Interval (also known as the AV-Delay) is the period of time that may elapse after a paced or sensed atrial event before a ventricular impulse will be delivered (Fig. 4.1). Under most circumstances an intrinsic QRS sensed before the end of the AVI will inhibit the ventricular output and the timing cycle will be reset for the next atrial output. The intrinsic event may be a normally conducted QRS due to intact AV-node function or it may be a PVC or premature junctional beat. Once a P-wave is sensed or an atrial stimulus is delivered, atrial sensing for the purpose of tracking P-waves is turned off until after the ventricular event occurs.

Differential AV Interval

Differential AVI is an enhancement of the basic AVI timer. It is known that the atrial contraction must be timed properly relative to the ventricular contraction to allow optimal preload and valve positioning in the ventricles. The timing is disrupted when a dual chamber pacemaker is in place. This is because when the pacemaker responds to a sensed P-wave the atrial depolarization is well underway. In contrast, when the device is pacing the atrium it is initiating the atrial contraction. In order to compensate for this difference, a different delay is allowed for paced and sensed atrial events before the ventricular output is delivered. The AVI following a sensed P-wave is allowed to be shorter than the AVI following a paced P-wave (Fig. 4.2). Some devices have a fixed nonprogrammable setting in the range of 25-50 msec. Other devices give many options for programming the difference between the two. In all devices the sensed AVI is shorter than the paced AVI. The result is a small but significant improvement in cardiac output.

Fig. 4.1. AV interval: The period of time in milliseconds between the paced or sensed atrial event until the paced ventricular event. If a sensed ventricular event occurs before the end of the AVI, the ventricular output will be withheld.

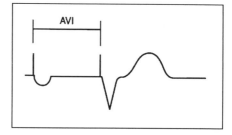

Fig. 4.2. Differential AV interval: The paced AVI is longer than the sensed AVI.

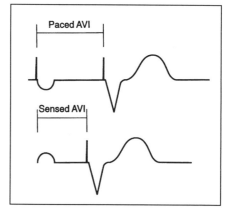

ADAPTIVE AVI

In a normally functioning heart the PR interval is not static. It varies with adrenergic tone and the heart rate. The PR interval shortens as the heart rate increases to continue providing optimal preload. Most newer dual chamber pacemakers now offer a feature known as adaptive AVI. As the name suggests, the AVI adapts based on the heart rate. Faster heart rates cause a shortening of the AVI (Fig 4.3). This results in two benefits. The first is more optimal hemodynamics for the patient by preserving the natural change in timing between atrium and ventricle. The second will become apparent when you learn about the total atrial refractory period and it's effect on the upper rate that the pacemaker can achieve. A shorter AVI will allow the pacemaker to operate normally at higher rates by allowing atrial sensing to occur at these higher rates.

ATRIAL ESCAPE INTERVAL (AEI)

The AEI is the maximum period of time that can elapse between the last sensed or paced ventricular event and the next atrial event. In ventricular based timing systems the AEI begins at any sensed or paced ventricular event (Fig. 4.4). It may be a sensed R-wave or a ventricular pacemaker pulse. If no intrinsic atrial beat occurs by the end of the AEI an atrial pace output will be delivered. The AEI may

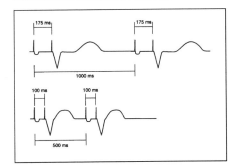

Fig. 4.3. Adaptive AVI interval: The AVI (both paced and sensed) will shorten as the pacing rate increases. In this example the AVI is 175 ms when the pacing rate is 60 bpm. The AVI shortens (usually in a gradual manner) to 100 ms when the pacing rate is 120 bpm.

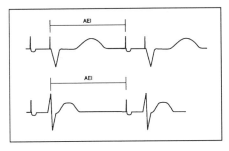

Fig. 4.4. Atrial escape interval: The amount of time that is allowed to elapse after a paced or sensed ventricular event, until the next atrial pace output will be delivered (unless an intrinsic P wave is sensed first).

be calculated by subtracting the AVI from the base pacing interval. For example, if the base pacing rate is 60 bpm this is a pacing interval of 1000 msec. An AVI of 200 msec would result in an AEI of 800 msec. It may also be determined by placing a pair of calipers on an atrial pace artifact and tracking back to the previous R-wave or ventricular pace artifact. Because of the variability of timing with R-wave sensing, it is most accurate when mapped back to the pace artifact.

POSTVENTRICULAR ATRIAL REFRACTORY PERIOD (PVARP)

PVARP is an atrial refractory period that begins following a paced or sensed ventricular event (Fig. 4.5). It serves two purposes. It turns off the atrial amplifier to prevent the atrial lead from sensing the ventricular depolarization (R-wave and T-wave) which could otherwise be misinterpreted by the pacemaker. It also prevents sensing of retrograde P-waves should a PVC occur. If the ventricle depolarizes before the atrium the electrical impulse may travel up the AV-node and cause an atrial contraction shortly **after** the ventricular contraction. This is not desired as the hemodynamics are poor and the patient's blood pressure may fall significantly. This may result in weakness and a number of other symptoms that together represent an entity known as pacemaker syndrome. In this situation the late atrial contraction may be sensed by the atrial lead and start the AV-interval timer again. The ventricle will be stimulated at the end of the AV-interval and the retrograde cycle will be started again (see section on Pacemaker Mediated Tachycardia in chapter 11). One of the more common methods of preventing this cycle from continuing is by programming the PVARP long enough that the retrograde

Fig. 4.5. Postventricular atrial refractory period (PVARP): An atrial refractory period occurs after each paced or sensed ventricular event.

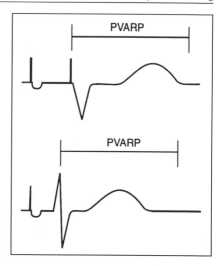

P-wave falls in this refractory period. The retrograde event will not be sensed and the cycle will not perpetuate. PVARP is often divided into two segments. The first portion is an absolute refractory period during which no sensing at all occurs. The second is a relative refractory period during which sensing may occur. Sensed events in the relative refractory period will not start an AVI. These events are used to enhance the diagnostic and therapeutic features such as automatic mode switching in dual chamber devices. The absolute portion of the PVARP is often referred to as the atrial blanking period. The PVARP minus the atrial blanking period is the relative refractory period.

TOTAL ATRIAL REFRACTORY PERIOD (TARP)

Since no atrial sensing for the purpose of tracking P-waves occurs during the AVI and the PVARP, the combination of the two adjacent intervals is referred to as the Total Atrial Refractory Period (AVI + PVARP = TARP). An atrial event occurring during TARP will not start another AVI and therefore cannot be tracked by the pacemaker. The TARP limits the upper rate limit of the pacemaker (see below). An easy way to remember the concept of TARP is to think of what happens when you put a "tarp" or tarpaulin over something; you can't see it.

ADAPTIVE PVARP

The limitations imposed upon the timing cycles by programming a longer PVARP may be substantial. It became apparent that a long PVARP is not needed all of the time. These limitations have been recently overcome to a great degree by allowing the PVARP to shorten or adapt with higher pacing rates. This feature is becoming more widely available in pacemakers that are sensor-driven. The pacemaker can use the data from the sensor to shorten the PVARP during periods of high metabolic need when higher heart rates are expected. This will allow the

TARP to shorten and allow higher tracking rates without the development of upper rate behavior. The PVARP remains longer at rest when it would be less likely that high atrial rates would be normal. Adaptive PVARP provides protection against retrograde conduction at rest and allows the shortened PVARP (and thus TARP) with exercise, permitting higher tracking rates.

UPPER RATE LIMIT (URL)

The URL is also referred to as the Maximum Tracking Rate (MTR) or the Maximum Tracking Interval (MTI). This is a programmable feature that limits the maximum rate (or shortest interval) at which the pacemaker will allow the ventricle to pace. If the atrial rate exceeds this limit either pacemaker Wenckebach or 2:1 (or higher degree) AV block will occur (see section on Upper Rate Behavior). The URL is programmable but is limited by the programmed TARP (remember that the TARP=PVARP+AVI). The longer the TARP the lower the allowable URL (Fig. 4.6). This is because atrial sensing is not present during TARP; therefore any P-waves falling into this combined period cannot be tracked. The URL may be separately programmable for tracking P-waves and for the upper sensor-driven rate.

BLANKING PERIOD

The blanking period is a brief ventricular refractory period that follows immediately after an atrial pulse is delivered. The purpose of this refractory period is to prevent the ventricular sensing channel from sensing the large atrial pulse. A normal ventricular sensitivity setting is in the range of 2 mV meaning that any electrical signal greater than 2 mV will inhibit the ventricular output. The atrial output pulse is commonly programmed between 2.5 and 5.0 V (that is 2500 to 5000 mV). It is easy to see how the ventricular channel could sense the atrial output and assume it saw a QRS. The ventricular output pulse will be inhibited and the patient will not have a ventricular beat. This problem is referred to as "crosstalk."

Fig. 4.6. Examples of URL calculation.

Example 1:

PVARP=300ms + AVI=200ms: TARP=500ms

Using the "Rule of 60,000"

60,000/500 = 120bpm highest programmable URL

Example 2:

PVARP=250ms + AVI=150ms: TARP=400ms

Using the "Rule of 60,000"

60,000/400 = 150bpm highest programmable URL

The blanking period is usually set in the range of 20-50 msec. Long blanking periods are very effective against crosstalk but limit the ability of the pacemaker to sense normal or premature ventricular beats. An additional discussion of this concept is found in the chapter on pacemaker malfunction.

Figure 4.7 shows a representation of the different timing mechanisms just discussed. It is important to remember that there is interaction between many of these parameters such that a change in one will affect one or more of the others.

ATRIAL BASED TIMING

The difference between ventricular based timing and atrial based timing relates to when the AEI begins after a sensed ventricular event. The two operate identically when the ventricle is being paced. As described above, in ventricular based timing the AEI will restart when a sensed ventricular beat occurs. However, this may have the effect of accelerating the pacing rate. As can be seen in Figure 4.8, the effect is rather small at slow rates. At high atrial pacing rates the difference can be significant and even cause violation of the URL. To prevent this from happening devices have been developed that use the so-called "atrial based" timing method. The purpose is to assure that the atrial pacing rate does not exceed the programmed URL. When an R-wave is sensed before the end of the AVI, and atrial based device does not begin the next AEI as would a ventricular based device. The atrial based device will wait until the programmed AVI would have terminated if no R-wave were detected. It then begins the next AEI and preserves the integrity of the entire pacing cycle (Fig. 4.9). In this way the next atrial output occurs when it should and is not accelerated.

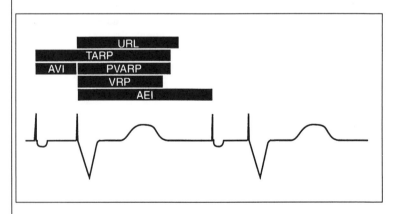

Fig.4.7. Dual Chamber Summary: This diagram summarizes and demonstrates the relationship between the major timing cycles; AVI, AEI, PVARP, TARP, URL. Note that the AVI + PVARP = TARP.

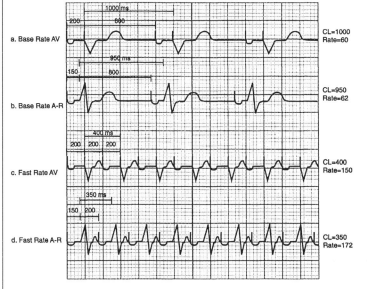
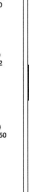

Fig. 4.8. Ventricular Based timing at low and high rates in a DDDR pacemaker with a lower rate of 60 bpm and an upper rate of 150 bpm. The AVI for pacing and sensing is 200. a. At the base pacing rate of 60 with AV pacing, the interval between QRS complexes is 1000 ms (60 bppm) as expected. b. In a patient with intrinsic AV-node function, the QRS occurs prior to the end of the AVI resulting in AR pacing. This starts the next AEI early resulting in a shortening of the interval between the QRS complexes by 50 ms in this example. The AEI begins 50 ms early, and this advances the next atrial output. At low rates this does not change the pacing rate significantly, with an increase of 2 bpm (to 62 bpm) in this example. c. At a sensor driven rate of 150 and AV pacing present, the actual pacing rate is 150 as would be expected. d. With intrinsic AV-node function as in exmaple (b), the QRS again occurs before the end of the AVI. The shortening of the AV interval of 50 ms now results in a pacing rate of 172 bpm, significantly higher than the maximum programmed rate.

DUAL CHAMBER PACING MODES

DDD MODE

There are many permutations of dual chamber pacing. The most widely used at this time is the DDD mode, also known as "universal" pacing mode. This provides Dual chamber pacing, Dual chamber sensing, and Dual mode of response to sensed events. The dual mode of response allows the device to be inhibited by sensed events (one mode of response) or to be triggered by a sensed event (second mode of response). The triggering occurs when a sensed atrial event starts an AVI followed by a paced ventricular event. This feature, also known as "tracking", maintains atrial-ventricular synchrony.

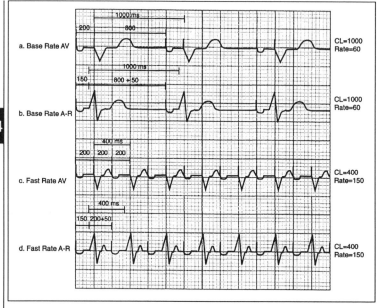

Fig. 4.9. Atrial Based timing at low and high rates. a. At the base pacing rate of 60 with AV pacing, the interval between QRS complexes is 1000 ms (60 bpm) as with ventricular based timing (see Fig. 4.8). b. In a patient with intrinsic AV-node function, the QRS occurs prior to the end of the AVI resulting in AR pacing. Unlike ventricular based timing, the AEI does not start when the QRS is sensed. The AEI starts after adding the rest of the time that was lost during the AVI (in this case an additional 50 ms). No change is seen in the base pacing rate which remains at 60 bpm. c. At a sensor driven rate of 150 and AV pacing present, the actual pacing rate is 150 as would be expected, and does not differ from that of ventricular based timing. d. With intrinsic AV-node function as in example (b), the QRS again occurs before the end of the AVI. The shortening of the AV interval of 50 ms is compensated for by adding back the "lost" 50 ms. The correct cycle length continues to be maintained, resulting in pacing at 150 bpm without violating the upper rate limit.

A pacemaker programmed to the DDD mode may appear on the ECG in any of four ways. The function may change from beat to beat as the patient's sinus rate and AV conduction vary.

The description of the cardiac events are often expressed as AS, AP, VS, VP to represent atrial-sensed, atrial-paced, ventricular-sensed and ventricular-paced events respectively. The method that will be used here is also common. P will indicate a sensed P-wave, R = a sensed R-wave; A = a paced atrial event and V = a paced ventricular event.

TOTALLY INHIBITED (PR)
This is seen when the intrinsic atrial rate is faster than the lower rate limit and AV-nodal conduction is more rapid than the programmed A-V delay. No pace artifact will be seen (Fig. 4.10).

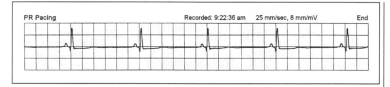

Fig. 4.10. PR pacing. Both the atrial and ventricular outputs are inhibited. The programming of this device was DDD with a lower rate limit of 45 and AVI of 230 ms.

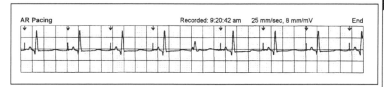

Fig. 4.11. AR pacing. The atrium is paced, but the AV node conducts the impulse to the ventricle before the end of the programmed AVI, inhibiting the ventricular output. This device was programmed DDD with a lower rate of 80 and an AVI of 230 ms. Note that the PVC resets the entire timing cycle.

ATRIAL PACE / VENTRICULAR INHIBITED (AR)

Only the atrial artifact will be seen followed by the patient's own QRS. This occurs when the intrinsic atrial rate is slower than the lower rate limit, and AV-nodal conduction is normal allowing the patients own QRS to occur before the end of the programmed AVI (Fig 4.11).

ATRIAL INHIBITED, VENTRICULAR PACE (PV)

Ventricular pacing will follow each intrinsic P-wave. This is seen when the intrinsic atrial rate is faster than the lower rate limit and is often referred to as tracking. The atrial output is inhibited due to the faster atrial rate. Only ventricular pacing is seen since the AV-nodal conduction is either not present or takes longer than the programmed AVI allows to occur (Fig 4.12).

ATRIAL-PACED AND VENTRICULAR PACED (AV)

Both atrial and ventricular pace artifacts will be present. This will be seen when the intrinsic atrial rate is slower than the lower rate limit and the patient's AV-nodal conduction is either not present or takes longer to conduct than the programmed AVI would allow (Fig 4.13).

DVI MODE

DVI provides Dual chamber pacing, but senses only in the Ventricle. Since there is no atrial sensing the triggering of a ventricular response by intrinsic atrial activity (tracking) is not possible. Since only ventricular sensing is present the only mode of response is to a ventricular sensed event. This will cause Inhibition of the ventricular output. If the atrial output has not yet occurred it is inhibited as well. This mode was common before DDD was available and is not commonly used now. It is still available as a programmed mode on many DDD pacemakers. DVI may be seen in a functional sense when the atrial lead loses it ability to sense in a device programmed to DDD. DVI may exist in two forms:

1) Committed: Once the device delivers an atrial impulse it will ALWAYS deliver a ventricular impulse even if an intrinsic R-wave occurs after the atrial pace (Fig. 4.14). This is often misinterpreted as pacemaker malfunction with ventricular under-sensing. Though this wastes energy it does provide complete protection against crosstalk (ventricular oversensing and inhibition by the atrial pace output-see chapter 11).

2) Noncommitted: The pacemaker will be inhibited as would be expected by an intrinsic R-wave, even if it has delivered an atrial output (Fig 4.15).

DDI MODE

This is a nontracking mode as is DVI. It provides Dual chamber pacing, Dual chamber sensing, but only Inhibition on a sensed event. The operation is similar

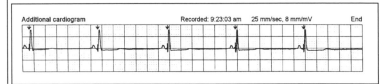

Fig. 4.12. PV pacing. The atrium is inhibited by the intrinsic P-wave and pacing occurs in the ventricle because it has not depolarized prior to the end of the programmed AVI. This device was programmed to DDD with a lower rate of 45 and an AVI of 170 ms.

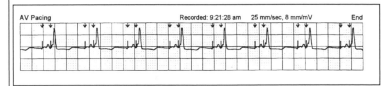

Fig. 4.13. AV pacing. Both the atrium and the ventricle are paced. This device was programmed to DDD with a lower rate of 80 and an AVI of 170 ms.

Fig. 4.14. DVI-C (committed) mode will pace both atrium and ventricle but sense only the ventricle. P waves are never sensed resulting in competition with native P-waves. Total inhibition of both atrial and ventricular output occurs only when a QRS is sensed before the end of the AEI. In this variation of DVI, any time an atrial output is delivered a ventricular output is "committed" as is seen on the third ARS. This "committed" operation is frequently mistaken for undersensing of the ventricular lead.

to DVI except that there is atrial sensing. Therefore, an intrinsic atrial event will inhibit the atrial output (Fig. 4.16). Since this will reduce or eliminate pacing shortly after a P-wave it is less likely to cause atrial arrhythmias. A device programmed to DDI cannot track the atrial rhythm. It will pace the atrium when the patient's atrial rate is lower than the programmed pacing rate. It will also pace the ventricle when the patient's ventricular rate is slower than the programmed rate. If the intrinsic atrial rate exceeds the programmed lower rate (due to sinus tachycardia, SVT, atrial flutter or atrial fibrillation), the atrial channel is inhibited and the pacemaker essentially functions in the VVI mode until the patient's atrial rate drops to the programmed rate. A comparison of DDD, DVI and DDI modes is shown in Figure 4.17. This is a very useful mode for patients with the diagnosis of sick sinus syndrome, carotid sinus hypersensitivity and bradycardia tachycardia syndrome. It is a poor choice in patients who have sustained or intermittent AV-block and normal sinus node function as it will not allow the pacemaker to maintain AV synchrony.

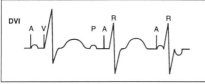

Fig. 4.15. DVI-NC (noncommitted) mode will pace both atrium and ventricle but sense only the ventricle. As with DVI-C, P waves are never sensed. Total inhibition of both atrial and ventricular output occurs only when a QRS is sensed before the end of the AEI. In this variation of DVI, the ventricular output is NOT committed after an atrial output. A QRS will inhibit the ventricular output at anytime up to the end of the AVI.

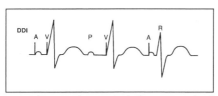

Fig. 4.16. DDI mode will pace and sense both atrium and ventricle. This eliminates the competition with intrinsic atrial beats as seen with the second P wave. The P wave is sensed and inhibits the atrial output, but does not start an AVI as would happen in a DDD system. The ventricular output will occur at the proper time to maintain the programmed pacing rate.

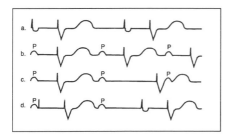

Fig. 4.17. Comparison of DDD, DDI and DVI: a. When atrial rates are slower than the base rate, DDD, DDI and DVI operate in an identical fashion. b. DDD: P-wave is sensed, starts an AVI and is tracked. c. DDI: P-wave is sensed and inhibits the atrial output, but does not start an AVI. The ventricular ouput occurs to maintain the base pacing rate. d. DVI: P-wave is not sensed at all. The paced atrial event is delivered at the end of the AEI, and the ventricular output at the end of the AVI. This results in competition between intrinsic and paced P-waves.

VDD MODE

This provides <u>V</u>entricular pacing, <u>D</u>ual chamber sensing and a <u>D</u>ual mode of response. Though a DDD device may be programmed to VDD, dedicated VDD devices are becoming increasingly popular. The latter have the advantage of using a single lead that is placed into the ventricle to pace and sense that chamber, with an extra electrode on the same lead that is capable of sensing but not pacing the atrium. VDD allows the atrium to be sensed and tracked for patients with complete AV-block (Fig 4.18). The disadvantage of VDD is that if the patient's heart rate falls below the lower rate limit of the pacemaker, pacing will be VVI as there is no capability to pace the atrium. VDD pacemakers will also exhibit upper rate response behavior (2:1 and Wenckebach) and may also allow pacemaker-mediated tachycardia (PMT).

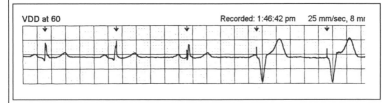

Fig. 4.18. VDD mode. This mode will sense the atrium and ventricle, but can only pace the ventricle. As the patient's heart rate slows, the device will transition from tracking the atrium to VVI pacing the ventricle. This can result in pacemaker syndrome due to a loss of AV synchrony. This mode is useful only for patients with normal SA node function and AV block.

Upper Rate Behavior
in Dual Chamber Pacing

5

INTRODUCTION

"Upper rate" behavior is intrinsic to the DDD and VDD pacing modes. It may be seen any time a mode is used that allows the ventricle to be paced as the result of an atrial-sensed event. Upper rate behavior occurs when the patient's atrial rate is faster than the programmed upper rate limit (URL) and/or exceeds the atrial sensing limits imposed by the programmed total atrial refractory period (TARP). Since a dual chamber pacemaker acts as an artificial AV-node, it is not surprising that the upper rate response is similar to AV-node behavior. When the patient's atrial rate reaches the limits imposed by the pacemaker in a patient with AV block one of two types of responses can be seen. These responses will not be seen in patients with normal AV node function as their own AV node will prevent the effects of this pacemaker behavior from becoming apparent.

2:1 BLOCK (MULTIBLOCK)

This would appear in much the same way as second degree (Mobitz-II) AV-block. 2:1 pacemaker block will occur when the maximum tracking rate is set to the limits imposed by the TARP (PVARP + AVI). For example, if the AVI is 200 msec and the PVARP is 300 msec, the TARP is 500 msec. Using the "Rule of 60,000" we can calculate that 500 msec is equal to 120 bpm. A pacemaker with these settings and the URL programmed to 120 bpm will exhibit 2:1 block behavior. This is also referred to as multiblock as higher degrees of block are possible. In this situation the patient's ventricular rate increases with the atrial rate until the URL is reached. Once the patient's atrial rate exceeds the URL every other P-wave will fall into the PVARP and is thus not sensed. As shown in Figure 5.1, 2:1 block then occurs and the patient's ventricular rate falls abruptly, often with significant symptoms. As the patient's atrial rate slows below the URL, the pacemaker will resume tracking the atrium and pace the ventricle 1:1 again.

Handbook of Cardiac Pacing, by Charles J. Love. © 1998 Landes Bioscience

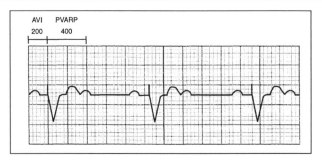

Fig. 5.1. 2:1 block will occur in a dual chamber pacing system when the interval between P-waves is shorter than the TARP. In this example the TARP is 600 ms creating a 2:1 block rate of 100 bpm. Once the atrial rate exceeds 100 bpm, P-waves begin to fall into the PVARP and are not sensed. This usually occurs abruptly (especially when the upper tracking rate is set to the same rate where 2:1 block will occur), causing significant symptoms for the patient.

PSEUDO-WENCKEBACH

This appears like classic Mobitz-I or Wenckebach block (Fig. 5.2). Pacemaker pseudo-Wenckebach behavior will occur rather than 2:1 type block when the URL is programmed to a rate lower than the limits imposed by the TARP. Using the example above with a TARP of 500 limiting the upper tracking rate to 120, programming a URL to 100 would result in Wenckebach behavior for atrial rates that exceed the URL of 100 bpm but are below the 2:1 block rate of 120 bpm. The difference between these two rates is referred to as the Wenckebach interval. It is preferable to program a device so that Wenckebach behavior will occur prior to the 2:1 block behavior. This allows the patient some warning before the heart rate drops abruptly. Though the symptoms are not as severe as in 2:1 block, the transient changes in ventricular preload and the intermittent failure to track the atrium 1:1 can be felt by most patients.

During the Wenckebach interval the P-waves ARE sensed as they do not fall during the refractory period. The pacemaker delays the ventricular output to prevent pacing the ventricle faster than allowed by the programmed URL. Should the pacemaker pace at the end of the programmed AVI the ventricular rate would exceed the URL. Because the ventricular output is delayed the AVI appears prolonged giving a Wenckebach appearance. Each successive AVI will lengthen until a P-wave falls into the atrial refractory period. Since this last P-wave cannot be tracked the following ventricular output is "dropped" and the cycle starts over again. If the atrial rate continues to rise and exceeds the atrial sensing limit imposed by the TARP, then 2:1 block will occur.

Several other methods have been developed to minimize the effect of abrupt onset 2:1 blocking:

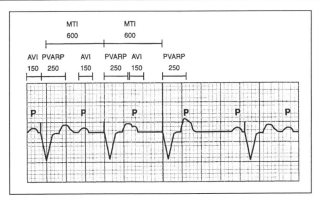

Fig. 5.2. Psudo Wenckebach behavior occurs when the upper tracking rate of the pacemaker is set lower than the 2:1 block rate (as determined by TARP). The appearance of the cardiogram will be identical to that of a patient with Mobitz-I AV-block. As a P wave is sensed at an interval shorter than allowed by the upper tracking rate, the ventricular output is delayed so as not to violate the upper rate limit. This results in an apparent prolongation of the AVI. This sequence continues until a P-wave falls within the PVARP and is therefore not sensed. This P wave will not start an AVI, and thus the next QRS is "dropped". The cycle will continue until the atrial rate drops below the upper rate limit at which time 1:1 conduction will resume.

RATE SMOOTHING

This is a feature available on some dual chamber pacemakers that limits changes in R to R intervals to a percentage of the previous interval. For example, by setting this parameter to a value of 6%, one cardiac cycle will not be allowed to differ from the previous one by more or less than 6% of the cycle length. By minimizing the beat to beat differences in cardiac cycles the effects of 2:1 block and pseudo-Wenckebach behavior are minimized. Figure 5.3 shows how this would appear. This feature may also be useful to reduce the pauses seen in patients with frequent PVCs and to reduce the risk of tracking retrograde atrial beats.

FALLBACK RESPONSE

This is a useful feature in patients that develop atrial arrhythmias as well as those who might have 2:1 upper rate behavior. Fallback allows the pacemaker rate to gradually decrease after the upper rate is reached. By doing this, 2:1 block does not result in an abrupt decrease in rate. In addition, should atrial fibrillation or flutter occur exceeding the URL, the pacemaker will gradually reduce the rate to the lower rate limit. This will stay in effect until the atrial rate drops below the

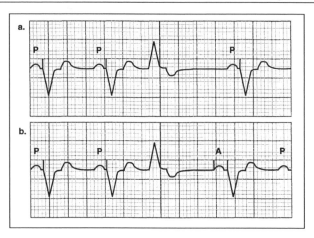

Fig. 5.3. Rate smoothing prevents one cardiac cycle length from differing from the previous cycle length by more than a percentage of the previous cycle. Tracing (a) shows a DDD pacemaker programmed to a lower rate of 60 without rate smoothing. In this example a PVC occurs resulting in a pause. Tracing (b) shows the response of the same pacemaker with rate smoothing enabled causing the pacemaker to reduce the effect of the premature beat by pacing earlier than would be expected.

URL at which time the pacemaker will resume tracking the atrium. Fallback response is usually programmable as to the rate to which it will fall and the period of time it will take to get to the fallback rate.

SENSOR-DRIVEN RATE SMOOTHING

Sensor-driven pacemakers are unique in that the lower rate limit changes based on a parameter other than the atrial rate. This feature is discussed in detail in chapter 6. The response of a DDDR pacemaker to an atrial rate that would normally cause 2:1 or Wenckebach behavior is essentially the same as that for a DDD device. The difference is that instead of the rate dropping to the programmed lower rate limit, the rate will drop to the sensor indicated rate at that time. This is referred to as "sensor-driven rate smoothing." For example, a patient has a DDDR pacemaker programmed to an upper rate and 2:1 block rate of 120 bpm. If the patient is running and the sensor rate indicates a minimum pacing rate of 115 bpm while the atrial rate is 125 bpm, the device will act as if the lower rate limit is 115. The pacing rate will vary between the URL of 120 and the sensor indicated rate of 115 until the native atrial rate falls below the URL. At that time 1:1 tracking of the atrial rate will resume. By preventing abrupt changes in paced rate the sensor has "smoothed" out the rhythm.

Sensor-Driven Pacing

INTRODUCTION

6

When the first pacemaker was implanted in 1958, pacemakers were used primarily in patients with compete AV-block. The devices were literally lifesaving for these patients. As pacemakers have improved and the patient population has changed, more patients now receive implants for sinus node disease than for AV-block. This is due to the aging population as well as the widespread use of beta blockers, calcium channel blockers, and anti-arrhythmia drugs such as sotalol and amiodarone. More recently the use of radiofrequency catheter ablation techniques as applied to patients with chronic atrial fibrillation has created a population of patients unable to adjust their own heart rates appropriately. The importance of proper heart rate response becomes apparent on review of the cardiac output equation:

Cardiac Output = Heart Rate x Stroke Volume

In patients with normal cardiac contractility the stroke volume increases to its maximal point when only 40% of maximal exertion has been achieved. Thus, increasing the heart rate is important during exercise to achieve the peak cardiac output. Patients with a fixed stroke volume such as those with dilated cardiomyopathy are not able to effectively increase their cardiac output by changes in contractility. They must rely entirely on changes in heart rate to increase the cardiac output.

The need to change the paced rate in proportion to metabolic demands has become essential in pacing to normalize the hemodynamic response as much as is possible. Patients unable to change their heart rates to meet metabolic demands are said to have "chronotropic incompetence." This may be an absolute or relative problem. A person who has atrial fibrillation and complete AV-block would have absolute chronotropic incompetence. For patients with chronotropic incompetence the use of standard DDD, VVI or AAI pacemakers does not provide the dynamic rate changes that are needed. Therefore, artificial sensors have been developed to compensate for this lack of normal heart rate response that the healthy sinus node normally provides.

There have been many sensors proposed and investigated (Table 6.1). The following discussion of the sensors will be limited to those in common clinical use.

ACTIVITY/VIBRATION

This method of adjusting the pacing rate by using a sensor was the first to be approved by the United States Food and Drug Administration. A piezoelectric crystal that generates an electrical signal when vibrated or stressed is bonded to the inside of the pacemaker. When the patient walks the vibrations from the body are transmitted through the pacemaker causing an electrical output to be generated from the crystal (Fig 6.1). These vibrations usually occur during and in proportion to the patient's level of physical activity. The electrical output from the sensor is proportional to the vibrations. The response of the pacemaker to the

---

Table 6.1. Sensors

Vibration
Accelerometer
Minute ventilation
Respiratory rate
Central venous temperature
Central venous pH
QT interval
Pre-ejection period (by pressure or volume change in the RV)
Right ventricular dP/dt (change in pressure/change in time)
Right ventricular dV/dt (change in volume/change in time)
Right ventricular stroke volume
Mixed venous oxygen saturation
Right atrial pressure
Evoked response

Fig. 6.1. The output of a piezioelectric crystal is proportional to the vibration and activity of the patient. The more the patient moves, the more rapid and higher amplitude the signal from the sensor.

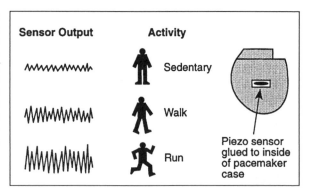

Sensor Output	Activity
	Sedentary
	Walk
	Run

Piezo sensor glued to inside of pacemaker case

body's vibration is adjusted by programming a threshold and slope value as well as a minimum and maximum rate. Other adjustments such as reaction and recovery time (also referred to as acceleration and deceleration time) may be available. The latest devices incorporate features to adjust some of these parameters automatically.

Simplicity is a major advantage of the vibration based systems. A standard implant technique, the use of standard unipolar or bipolar leads, a low current drain and the widespread use of this type of system are the strengths of activity sensors. Unfortunately vibration is not always proportional to metabolic need. Swimming and bicycle riding are two of the more common activities that vibration based devices do not handle well. Neither activity produces the same vibration and therefore sensor response that walking or running will produce. The response may be improved if the device is programmed to be more sensitive; however, it will then over respond to normal walking. Bicycle riders face the additional issue of paradoxical sensor responses. When a bicycle rider starts up a hill the pedaling rate slows and the vibrations decrease. This results in a slowing of the paced rate at a time when increased rate is needed. We have taught some of our bike riders to reach up with one hand and tap over the pacemaker to cause the sensor to increase the pacing rate. This technique may also be used for patients with orthostatic hypotension. Before the patient rises from the supine position they can tap on the pacemaker causing an increase in pacing rate. This helps to blunt the drop in blood pressure. There is also the potential for spurious responses. Loud music with a deep bass, riding in a car going down a bumpy road or even sleeping in a manner that puts pressure on the pacemaker will cause increased pacing rates. Certain occupations that expose the patient to severe vibration may also cause unwanted rate increases.

Programming a vibration device can be rather complex. In a device that does not have automatic features or programmer based algorithms to assist in setting these parameters one must adjust them all manually. On all sensor-driven pacemakers the first parameters that must be set are the lower and upper rate. Changing either of these after the other parameters are set may change the pacemaker response significantly. The next setting to be addressed is the sensor threshold. This sets the lowest level of output from the sensor that will cause the pacing rate to rise. Any signals from the sensor that exceed the threshold level will be counted and used to adjust the pacing rate (Fig. 6.2). Threshold settings may be numeric (lower numbers reflect a lower and more responsive threshold) or descriptive (such as low, medium and high). I prefer to have the patient take a walk down a hallway in a normal fashion and adjust the threshold so that at a reasonable sensor response occurs. If no sensor response occurs then the threshold is lowered. If an excessive response occurs the threshold is increased.

After the threshold is adjusted, the slope should be set. This parameter is responsible for the pacemaker reaching a desired rate for a given amount of activity. It may respond to the number of sensor "counts" that exceed the threshold value, or it may use the integral of the areas generated by the sensor activity above threshold (Fig 6.3). In either case, increasing the slope will result in an increased

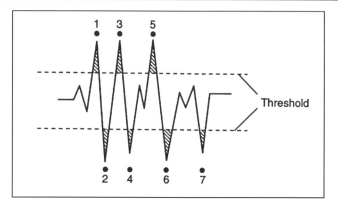

Fig. 6.2. This diagram represents signals from a piezoelectric sensor. Those that exceed the threshold are counted. Alternatively, the area that exceeds threshold (shaded) is determined.

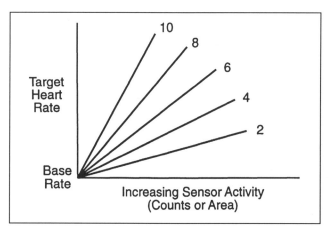

Fig. 6.3. Once the counts or integrated area of the sensor activity are determined, the slope value chosen will determine the target heart rate.

pacing rate for the same amount of activity. The response of the pacemaker to a given sensor output will also depend on the shape of the slope used in a particular pacemaker. Some use a linear algorithm while others use one that is curvilinear. A low slope using a curvilinear algorithm may not allow the paced rate to reach a programmed high upper rate even with maximum output of the sensor.

The use of a reaction and recovery time is necessary on vibration based devices. This is due to the fact that when the patient begins to walk the sensor response goes from zero to some increased value. One does not want the heart rate to "jump" to the target rate in just a couple of beats. The reaction/acceleration time allows a gradual increase in pacing rate to the new target rate. Conversely, when the patient stops, the vibration rate plummets to zero. Since it would not be physiologic for the heart rate to fall abruptly, a recovery/deceleration time is programmed to ease the rate down to the lower rate limit (Fig. 6.4). Though most patients do well with the "out of the box" settings, patients with poor cardiac output may benefit from faster reaction times and longer recovery times.

ACCELEROMETER

A variation on the vibration based systems is the accelerometer. These devices have all of the same features and advantages of the vibration based devices, but are less likely to have spurious responses. Though more responsive to movements other than walking and running than vibration based devices, the failure to respond appropriately to certain types of activities (such as bike riding) remains a problem. The programming of these devices is essentially the same as those with the vibration type of sensor. Figure 6.5 shows four types of accelerometer sensors. One type places a piezoelectric crystal on a "diving board platform" mounted on the circuit board rather than on the pacemaker case. This isolates the crystal from most vibration but allows it to be flexed by forward and backward motion. Another application using piezoelectric material places it between two weights. As the patient moves, the weights flex the material generating signals. A specialized chip has been devised that allows interposed fingers to move relative to each other with motion. This changes an electric field between them to provide motion detection. Finally, a small metal ball that moves within an elliptical chamber as the patient moves. This disturbs an electrical field and provides the necessary signals to adjust the pacing rate.

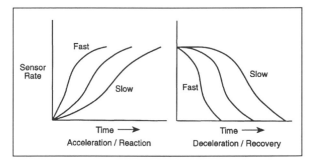

Fig. 6.4a. Acceleration time: Once the target heart rate is determined, the acceleration time will determine how quickly this new rate will be achieved. b. Deceleration time: When the activity is stopped, the deceleration time will determine long it will take the paced rate to return to the base rate.

Fig 6.5. Accelerometers. a. Platform mounted piezoelectric crystal. b. Cantilevered piezoelectric crystal. c. 3 layer silicon suspended bridge. d. Metal ball in an elliptical chamber.

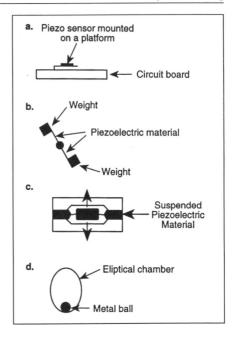

6

CENTRAL VENOUS TEMPERATURE

The first true metabolic sensor to be approved for use in the U.S. was based on measuring the blood temperature in the right ventricle. As the patient becomes physically active the muscle activity generates heat that warms the blood. As this blood returns to the central circulation a thermistor in the pacemaker lead senses the increase in temperature (Fig. 6.6). The pacing rate is then increased in proportion to the rise in temperature. A minimum and maximum rate are programmed as well as a slope and an intermediate rate. Additional parameters may require programming as well. Systems based on temperature are sometimes slow to respond due to an initial drop in blood temperature at the start of exertion. The drop is caused by blood that had been circulating slowly (and thus cooling) in the extremities returning to the heart at the onset of exercise. The cool returning blood will actually cause an initial drop in central venous blood temperature and will delay the sensor response. Newer algorithms have been developed to take advantage of the initial temperature drop to signal the onset of exercise. The drop will the pacemaker to increase its rate to the intermediate rate. It will then wait temperature begins to rise. If no rise occurs, the rate will revert back to limit. As seen in Figure 6.7, the drop is most pronounced in patients output. This can be explained by the vasoconstriction and cooler xtremities in these patients when at rest. Though this system arameter it may respond inappropriately to temperature

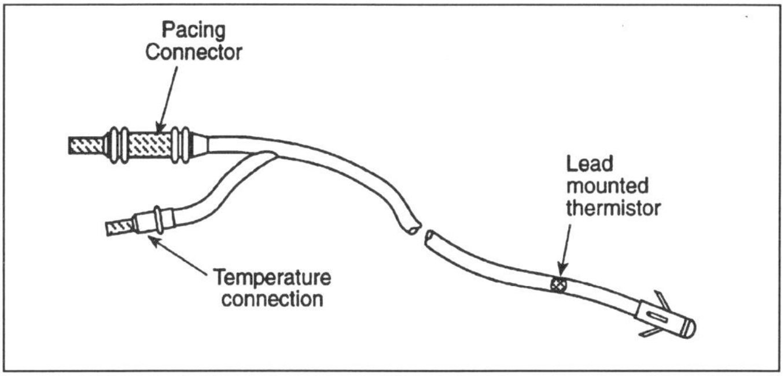

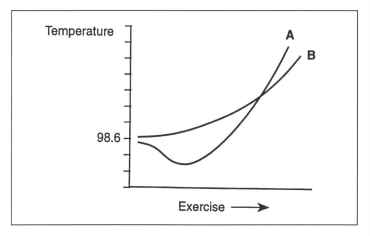

Fig. 6.6. In a specialized lead design, a thermistor is incorporated into the lead to detect small changes in right ventricular blood temperature. Note the additional connector on the lead.

6

Fig. 6.7. Graph of central venous temperature versus time with increasing exercise. With this type of system an increase in central venous temperature leads to increase in pacing rate. Curve A is of a patient with dilated cardiomyopathy and congestive heart failure showing initial drop in temperature as cool blood returns to the central circulation. Curve B is of a patient with a normal ventricle.

changes caused by fever, bathing, and drinking hot liquids. In addition, it requires a specialized sensor in the lead system. Reliability has not been as good as with devices where the sensor is based inside the pacemaker.

MINUTE VENTILATION (CHEST WALL IMPEDANCE CHANGE)

The detection of changes in respiratory rate and depth is becoming an increasingly popular metabolic parameter to use in pacing. Minute ventilation is closely related in a linear fashion to work rate and oxygen uptake. Pacemakers using minute ventilation as a sensor are capable of determining an approximation of minute ventilation using the technique of chest wall resistance measurement (thoracic impedance plethysmography). This technique uses small pulses of electrical current delivered between the pacemaker and the ring electrode (anode) of the lead (Fig. 6.8). In one system commonly used, the pulses are 1 mA in amplitude and 15 microseconds in duration. These are not strong enough or long enough to stimulate the heart. The pacemaker then measures the voltage changes between the pacemaker and the lead tip (cathode). The system uses the known amount of current delivered and the measured voltage to calculate changes in impedance (resistance) across the chest wall using a reformulation of Ohm's Law (Resistance = Volts/Current). The frequency of change in resistance is equal to the respiratory rate, and the degree of change is proportional to the tidal volume (Fig. 6.9). This yields an approximation of minute volume. As the minute volume increases the pacing rate increases proportionately. A minimum and maximum rate are set, as well as a slope (called the rate response factor in some of these systems). A reaction time may also be available as an option. The advantage of this type of system is the use of a true metabolic parameter to drive rate changes. The disadvantage is the need for a bipolar lead. The only contraindication for use of this sensor is its use in patients that can exceed 60 breaths per minute. This is seen only in the pediatric population, and rarely in adults with psychogenic hyperventilation syndrome. It is also not recommended for implants where the pacemaker is placed in an abdominal pocket. This type of sensor responds well to a wide variety of exercise and emotional demands as it is linked to a true metabolic parameter.

Fig. 6.8. Minute ventilation concept with lead and pacemaker. This system delivers a known amount of current (1 mA) between the ring electrode and the pacemaker case (pathway A). The voltage across the chest wall is then measured between the tip electrode and the pacemaker case (pathway B). The changes in resistance are calculated in accordance with Ohm's Law (see text).

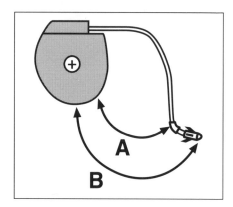

Fig. 6.9. Changes in chest wall resistance (impedance) are equal to the respiratory rate and proportional to the tidal volume.

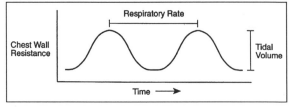

EVOKED Q-T INTERVAL

It is well known that as the heart rate increases that the QT interval will decrease. Indeed, we routinely correct the QT interval and report it as the QTc based on the heart rate. There is a second component to QT shortening that is based on the sympathetic state and the degree of catecholamine response. This second component of QT shortening is independent of the heart rate. Pacemakers using this concept to trigger an increase in pacing rate use the pace to T-wave interval. As the sympathetic tone increases in response to exercise the pace to T-wave interval decreases (Fig. 6.10). In response the pacemaker will increase the pacing rate. Conversely, as the pace to T-wave interval lengthens due to a decrease in sympathetic tone, the pacing rate will be lowered. This technique will respond not only to changes caused by exertion, but also to emotional changes. A patient who is in pain or is startled will experience an increase in paced rate. While this may be a physiologic response, it may not be desirable for the patient with ischemic heart disease and angina. There are several limitations of this type of device. First, in order to measure the pace to T-wave interval the device must pace intermittently, even if the native rate is faster than the sensor indicated rate. Second, it can only be used in the ventricle or in dual chamber systems. Stand alone atrial applications such as AAIR will not work as the device cannot operate without the ventricular lead. Third, it is possible for the algorithm to cause a "spiral" to the upper rate. This can occur due to the fact that faster pacing will cause a rate dependent shortening of the QT interval which will further increase the rate. Because of this possibility a feature called "nulling" is present in these devices. Nulling allows the device to return to the lower rate limit and recalibrate if the pacing rate remains elevated for an extended period of time. Nulling may be a limitation for patients who exercise for more than short periods of time.

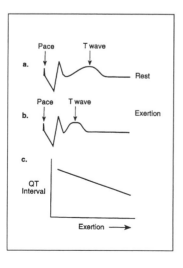

Fig. 6.10. With increasing catecholamines and/or sympathetic tone, the pace to T-wave interval shortens (a, b). This shortening occurs in proportion to exercise (c), resulting in the pacemaker increasing its paced rate.

MIXED VENOUS OXYGEN SATURATION

Though not in current use in a market-released pacemaker, this is an interesting and effective sensor. It utilizes a specialized pacing lead with a light emitting diode (LED) and a photodetector (Fig. 6.11). The LED delivers brief pulses of light in the right ventricular blood pool that are reflected back to the photodetector. The detector determines the color and thus the degree of oxygenation of the venous blood. As the oxygenation drops the paced rate increases (Fig 6.12). This is a very physiologic system, however reliability problems with the specialized lead have kept it from mainstream use.

There are many other sensors that are not in general use at this time. These have been listed in Table 6.1. The most important new concept in sensor-driven pacing is the use of more than one sensor to determine the need for a rate change. These pacemakers combine two sensors (e.g., activity with minute ventilation,

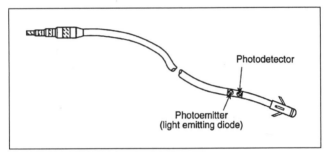

Fig. 6.11. A specialized lead for measuring the oxygen saturation in the right ventricle. A photoemitter (light emitting diode) is combined with a photodetector on the lead body. Note that a special quadrapolar lead is used with a 4 pole connector.

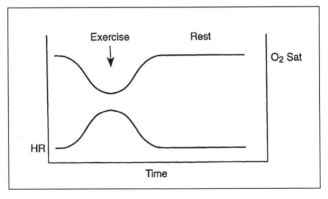

Fig. 6.12. As oxygen saturation in the venous system decreases with exertion, the pacing rate will be increased to match the workload.

QT with minute ventilation, temperature with activity, or QT and activity) to regulate the heart rate. The advantage of using a combination of sensors relates to combining the strengths of each sensor to overcome their individual shortcomings. Using the rapidly responding activity sensor with the slower but more physiologic minute ventilation sensor results in a fast and accurate system. Each sensor may also be used to check the accuracy of the other. Should one sensor indicate a need for rate increase to the maximal rate, yet the other indicate that the patient is at rest, the device may use the data of the more reliable sensor or recalibrate the system to limit the paced response. The dual sensor systems are just being introduced to the market at this time. They will provide additional challenges to properly program and follow two sensors instead of one.

I would like to emphasize the importance of programming the sensors properly for the individual patient. The vast majority of patients that we see have their pacemakers set to the nominal ("out of the box") settings. We find that this is not optimal for approximately 80% if the patients. It should only take two to five minutes to set the sensor properly, yet this is not routinely done by many physicians. The result is a device that paces either too slowly or too rapidly for any given level of patient activity. Patients are thereby limited or become symptomatic unnecessarily.

Advanced Pacemaker Features

As additional features and capabilities have been added to pacemakers the need for advanced therapeutic and diagnostic capability within the devices has grown. This chapter will explore these newer features and explain their function and use.

AV/PV HYSTERESIS

The AV interval has already been discussed with regard to differential and adaptive modification. The application of a hysteresis interval to the AVI may be done to provide consistent pacing of the ventricle or to prevent constant pacing of the ventricle.

POSITIVE AV INTERVAL HYSTERESIS

It has been shown by many investigators that a narrow nonpaced QRS achieves a greater stroke volume than a paced left bundle branch block pattern QRS. The rationale behind positive AVI hysteresis is to maintain a normal nonpaced QRS whenever possible. This provides an optimal contraction pattern and stroke volume. Positive AVI hysteresis adds an additional interval onto the programmed AVI for one cycle. If a sensed QRS occurs during this prolonged AV interval the device maintains the longer interval. If the device does not sense a QRS during the longer interval, pacing continues at the normal programmed AVI. It will check (or "search") for intrinsic conduction intermittently by inserting the extra interval (Fig 7.1). For this reason the term "autointrinsic conduction search" has been used to describe positive AVI hysteresis. I like to refer to this as "functional mode switching" as it allows the pacemaker to function as an AAI or AAIR system until loss of AV-conduction occurs. It then appears to switch back to DDD or DDDR functionality.

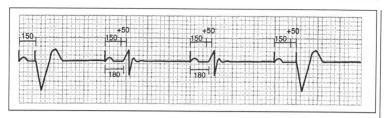

Fig. 7.1. Positive AV Iinterval Hysteresis (Auto Intrinsic Conduction Search). This feature is designed to allow intrinsic AV node conduction to occur whenever possible. During AV pacing, after 256 ventricular paced events the pacemaker will insert an extra period during the AV interval to search for intrinsic conduction. In this example the base AV interval is programmed to 150 ms, and the positive AV hysteresis is programmed to 50 ms. The second AV interval is a "search interval", and the QRS is conducted via the AV node. The pacemaker output to the ventricle is withheld due to the extra 50 ms added to the AV interval and the intrinsic conduction. On the last beat, the AV node fails to conduct and the pacemaker paces at the end of the extended interval. Following this beat the original programmed AV interval will be restored until the search occurs again 256 beats later. If during the "search" no intrinsic conduction is seen, the base AV interval is restored for the next 255 beats.

7

NEGATIVE AV INTERVAL HYSTERESIS

This feature works like positive AVI hysteresis except that it attempts to maintain a paced QRS at all times instead of a nonpaced QRS. The intention is to maintain the longest AV interval that results in a paced ventricular complex. There are some investigational data to suggest that this is beneficial in patients with hypertrophic obstructive cardiomyopathy. By maintaining a left bundle branch block pattern via early depolarization of the right ventricular apex, the intraventricular septum depolarizes later. This has the effect of reducing the outflow tract obstruction. The effect can be profound in some patients. However, one also wants to maintain the longest AVI that will allow this beneficial effect of early depolarization that allows the most ventricular filling time possible. Negative AV hysteresis works to shorten the AV interval if an intrinsic QRS is sensed before the end of the programmed AV interval. Once the AVI is shortened by this feature, it will be lengthened to the programmed AV interval intermittently to see if intrinsic conduction is still present. If an intrinsic QRS is sensed during this "search" beat, the shorter interval is maintained. If conduction is not present then the longer programmed AVI is restored (Fig. 7.2).

AUTOMATICITY

As pacing systems become more complex, programming the parameters to optimal values for each individual patient becomes more difficult. In addition, biological systems by their nature are constantly changing, making settings that are appropriate at one point in time inappropriate at some other time. Some pacemakers now have algorithms to automatically adjust one or more parameters.

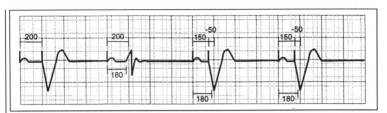

Fig. 7.2. Negative AV Interval Hysteresis attempts to maintain constant pacing of the ventricle. Any time a QRS is sensed after a P wave the AVI is shortened by a programmed amount which, in this example, is 50 ms. This feature is useful in patients with obbstructive hypertrophic cardiomyopathy.

Currently, automaticity is most commonly applied to the rate response sensor function. This allows the device to respond in a reasonable manner without significant intervention by the physician. In the vibration and accelerometer types of devices, an automatic threshold setting looks at the average amount of signal coming from the sensor during the previous day. Since the majority of time for virtually all patients is spent at rest, this provides a fairly accurate and very reproducible baseline for threshold. Any activity that produces sensor output exceeding this average threshold value will result in an increased pacing rate. An offset may be added to make the threshold higher or lower than the average as determined by the device, allowing some customization for each patient.

A similar automatic feature has been added to the rate response slope parameter. The pacemaker has a "picture" of a normal heart rate response stored in it's memory. Some devices have several of these pictures stored (normal, very active or sedentary) and one may be chosen that best fits the activity level of the particular patient. If the pacemaker sees that the heart rate response at the current slope setting is lower than expected, the slope will increase automatically. The opposite will occur if the sensor response appears to be excessive. This change in slope will occur slowly (for example one or two units per week), and it may be limited to a maximum change so that the automatic adjustment does not vary too far from the initial programmed setting.

There are algorithms to adjust the atrial and ventricular sensitivity of the pacemaker. I have found these to be somewhat less than useful. They often result in reducing the sensitivity of the device such that some PACs or PVCs are not sensed. There are several algorithms, and they are mostly complex and will not be discussed in this book. For a bipolar pacing system the nominal ("out of the box") settings for sensitivity are usually quite adequate and rarely result in under or over sensing. Pacemakers are now being designed with an automatic gain feature similar to that of implantable defibrillators. This differs from the automatic adjustment feature currently in use in that the programmed values are not affected (Fig. 7.3).

The most critical parameter to be adjusted automatically is the pacing output. This may be done by changing the amplitude, the duration of the pulse or both. The capture threshold is tested by the pacemaker on a regular basis (hourly, daily, weekly, etc.). The output is then adjusted to some value above the threshold value.

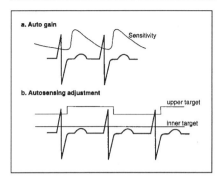

Fig. 7.3a. Auto Gain is a method of automating sensing function. The longer the device goes without sensing a signal the more sensitive it becomes. Once a signal is sensed, the sensitivity abruptly decreases to avoid oversensing the evoked response and the T wave. b. Autosensing adjustment is a method to automatically set the sensitivity of the pacemaker. An inner and upper target are set for sensing. When a beat is sensed on both the upper and inner targets, the upper target is moved further out (made less sensitive) until sensing no longer occurs. The upper target is then moved back in. In this way the device can determine the amplitude of the signals and set the overall sensitivity of the device appropriately.

By continuously adjusting the output to remain just a small increment above the threshold, significant current savings are possible while maintaining safety. This translates into much better pacemaker longevity. Another feature of some devices that have automatic output regulation is "capture confirmation." With this algorithm each individual pace output is checked for effective capture. If capture does not occur, a backup high output pulse is immediately delivered (Fig 7.4). Should more than one of these events occur consecutively, a threshold search is initiated and a new output level is set. This scheme provides both longevity and safety. Currently, capture confirmation is available only when using a bipolar lead. The output is delivered in a unipolar fashion from the tip of the lead to the pacemaker. The intracardiac signal is then seen on the ring electrode (anode) in a bipolar fashion.

AUTOMATIC MODE SWITCHING

A problem that has plagued dual chamber pacemakers for many years is the limitation imposed when utilizing the DDD or VDD based modes in patients with intermittent atrial tachyarrhythmias. When the patient develops atrial fibrillation, atrial flutter, or other supraventricular tachycardia, a standard DDD pacer "tracks" this rhythm and paces the ventricle to the programmed upper rate limit. Use of DDI or DVI can prevent this, but then a patient who also has AV-block cannot track the atrium during sinus rhythm. There are several approaches to allowing the pacemaker to actually change it's mode from DDD, DDDR, VDD or VDDR to either DDI, DDIR, VVI or VVIR. The mode that results from the switch is dependent on the initial programmed mode and the model of the pacemaker. Mode switching is especially useful in patients with AV block as they are in need of tracking the atrium when it is in sinus rhythm. Patients with intact AV node function and poor SA node function may be paced in the DDIR mode without compromise. This mode will allow atrial pacing when the patient is in sinus rhythm but will effectively pace VVIR when the atrial rate is high.

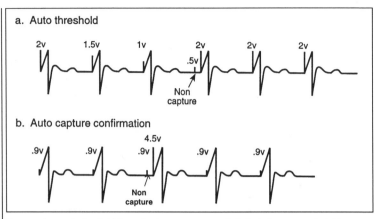

Fig. 7.4a. Automatic threshold determination occurs on a periodic basis (e.g., once a day). The output stimulus is reduced until capture no longer occurs. At this point a rescue pulse is delivered and the output of the pacemaker is reprogrammed to some value above the threshold value. b. Capture confirmation occurs on a beat to beat basis. Each output is evaluated for the presence of an evoked response. If no QRS occurs within the detection window, a high output resue pulse is delivered. This occurs so rapidly (<65 ms) that the patient is totally unaware that anything has happened.

DDDR devices can utilize the sensor to evaluate whether the atrial rhythm is appropriate (such as sinus tachycardia due to exercise) or inappropriate (such as atrial fibrillation) for a given level of activity. If a rapid atrial rate is seen and the sensor indicates that the patient is at rest, the event is classified as pathologic. The pacemaker then converts to VVIR until the atrial rate drops into the "physiologic range" again at which time DDDR function is restored.

Another approach that does not require a sensor is to simply use a separately programmable "atrial tachycardia detection rate" (or "mode switch rate"). If the atrial rate exceeds the detection rate for a given period of time or a specific number of beats, the device will switch to a nontracking mode. It will switch back when the atrial rate drops back into the normal range (Fig 7.5).

The newest feature introduced in an attempt to deal with atrial arrhythmias is known as Smart Tracking. This algorithm sets an upper rate for which the pacemaker will track the atrial rate. Atrial rates exceeding this upper rate result in mode switch or fallback to the sensor indicated rate. This algorithm will adjust this upper tracking rate in response to the patient's activity. The higher the sensor indicated rate, the faster the pacemaker is allowed to track the atrial rate. By adjusting this upper rate limit in response to the patient's activity, there is protection from atrial arrhythmias that is proportional to expected atrial rates. This works without limiting the upper rate response of the device.

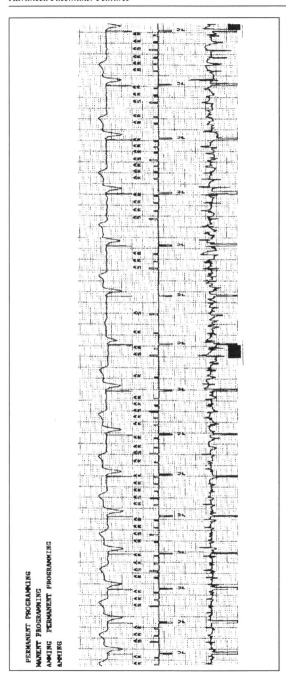

Fig. 7.5a. Automatic Mode Switching onset. This patient with a DDDR pacemaker (programmed to a lower rate of 60 and an upper tracking rate of 130) develops atrial fibrillation (note the atrial refractory sense markers—AR, and the atrial EGM on the bottom). The pacemaker initially tracks the fib to the upper rate, but then gradually falls to the lower programmed rate as it switches from DDD to VVI.

7

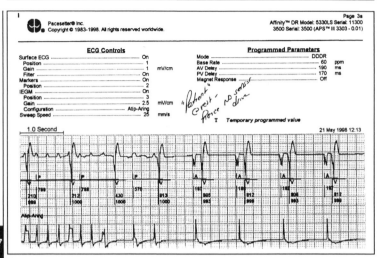

Fig. 7.5b. Automatic Mode Switching Offset. Once the atrial fibrillation terminates, the pacemaker resumes dual chamber pacing. Contributed by Dr. Paul Levine, M.D.

RATE DROP RESPONSE

Recent studies have shown an improved outcome by pacing patients who have autonomic dysfunction with a cardioinhibitory response alone or combined with a vasodepressor response. The rate drop response feature was designed specifically for this type of patient. The pacemaker is set with a lower pacing rate and a therapeutic pacing rate. It is also set with a heart rate zone and a rate of change within that zone. If the patient's heart rate falls abruptly through this detection zone, the pacemaker will begin to pace at the higher therapeutic rate for a specified amount of time (Fig. 7.6). This provides additional heart rate to counteract the drop in stroke volume, hopefully maintaining the cardiac output. If the patient's heart rate passes through this zone slowly, then the therapeutic response is not initiated. This prevents rapid pacing when the patient is at rest or sleeping.

SLEEP MODE / CIRCADIAN RESPONSE

It is routine to program the pacemaker to a lower rate limit in the range of 60-80 bpm. This is done to support the patient during the waking hours of the day. It is not physiologic to maintain these rates when sleeping. This is the rationale behind features designed to slow the rate during inactivity or sleep. The first method of accomplishing this goal was the use of an internal clock in the pacemaker. One can set the current time, the patient's normal waking time and normal bedtime. A separate sleep rate is then programmed to be in effect during the expected sleep time. If the patient gets up and becomes active during the desig-

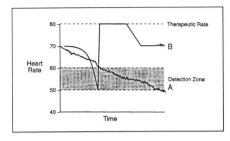

Fig. 7.6. Rate Drop Response is a feature that triggers a higher "therapeutic" pacing rate if the patient's own rate drops abruptly. Curve A shows a gradual slowing of the heart rate through the shaded detection zone. This would be typical of a person falling asleep. No therapeutic pacing would be delivered in this situation. Curve B shows an abruptly decreasing heart rate such as might be seen with carotid sinus hypersensitivity, or a "vasovagal" episode. When the detection zone is crossed rapidly like this, the pacemaker responds with pacing at a higher rate for a period of time, then falls back to its "ready state".

nated sleep time, the rate sensor notes the activity and overrides the sleep rate. This clock based algorithm works pretty well except for the fact that: 1) a patients sleep times may vary greatly, 2) patients may nap at odd hours during the day, 3) daylight savings time comes and goes but the device does not take this into account, and 4) patients and their pacemakers cross time zones but the internal pacemaker clock has no way of knowing this. A more recent iteration of this feature uses the variability of patient activity as determined by the rate modulation sensor. As the patient becomes inactive for a period of time, this is noted by the pacemaker. It will then allow the rate to drop to the sleep rate. As soon as the patient becomes active again, the pacemaker resumes the regular lower rate limit. This algorithm has the advantage of being patient based rather than clock based.

AUTOMATIC POLARITY CHANGE/LEAD MONITOR

One of the concerns regarding pacing is what happens when a lead breaks or the insulation fails. If a break occurs in a bipolar lead on the cathodal conductor coil, little can be done. However, if the break occurs on the anodal coil a pacemaker with programmable polarity may be reprogrammed to the unipolar configuration thus bypassing the failed coil. The same can be done if the lead impedance falls to a low level on a bipolar lead to prevent a "dead short" between the two coils. Automatic polarity switching is available on some pacemakers to provide this added measure of safety. The change in polarity occurs via one of two algorithms. The first uses abrupt changes in lead impedance as measured intermittently to trigger the change. The second uses a small unipolar electrical pulse down the anode after each cardiac cycle to look for electrical noise that is typically present with a conductor coil failure.

Many different diagnostic features are now available to assist in determining whether the pacemaker has been operating and responding appropriately. They are also quite useful to determine what the patient's heart rate and rhythm have been. The following is a review of the more common counters, trends and histograms that are widely used.

COUNTERS AND HISTOGRAMS

The simplest counters tell what percent of the time pacing is occurring or how many paced events have occurred since the last evaluation. In a VVI pacemaker placed in a patient with atrial fibrillation this counter may be used to determine the effectiveness of medical therapy being used to slow the AV node. If the percent paced is very low, the patient is likely having a faster than desired ventricular response as it is inhibiting the pacemaker most of the time. Figure 7.7 shows a more advanced counter that not only counts the number of paced and sensed events, but also classifies them based on the rate. This is a much more powerful tool to determine the effectiveness of medical therapy. When this same feature is applied to a dual chamber pacemaker it becomes a bit more complex. The device must now track pacing and sensing in both chambers, what percent of the time this occurs, and the functional state of the device for each event (Fig 7.8). This type of histogram is quite useful to evaluate the appropriateness of the programmed sensor and AVI values. In addition, a peak at a high rate in the atrial histogram may indicate a pathologic condition such as intermittent atrial fibrillation (Fig 7.9). The examples shown are representative, as every manufacturer has a unique way of presenting the data.

Fig. 7.7. Event histogram counts printout VVIR pacemaker shows the percent of time the device is pacing and sensing. This device also provides for a breakdown of the heart rates into ranges, and whether these were paced or sensed events. This may be useful to adjust medications that block the AV node, or to adjust the rate response sensor.

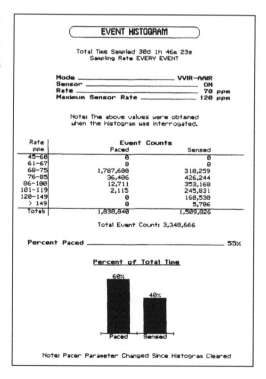

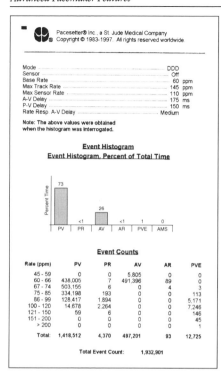

Fig. 7.8. Event histogram counts printout DDDR pacemaker. Not only does this show the heart rate ranges and percent paced, but it also provides a breakdown of the state of pacing at these times. This patient has complete AV-Block, and thus the majority of events are in the "PV" state. Atrial pacing (AV state) is seen only when the patient's sinus rate drops to the lower rate limit of the pacemaker.

7

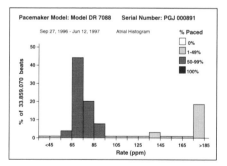

Fig. 7.9. This histogram was obtained from a device implanted in a patient with intermittent atrial fibrillation. Note that appproximately 20% of the atrial sensed events occur in the >185 range. This histogram is useful in determining whether medical therapy is effective in controlling the atrial rhythm.

The sensor indicated rate histogram evaluates the performance of the sensor. It is important to understand that this will indicate the rate that the pacemaker WOULD be pacing the heart if the patient were 100% paced (Fig. 7.10). If the patient's own heart rate exceeds the sensor indicated rate and inhibits the pacemaker, the histogram will underestimate the actual heart rate. This counter may also be used while the sensor is in a "passive" mode. It allows evaluation of sensor performance without actually pacing the patient at increasing heart rates. This is very useful when first programming the sensor to avoid pacing the patient at an excessively fast rate if the sensor is set too aggressively.

TRENDS

While histograms are very useful they present a lot of data lumped together. It is not possible to determine when an event happened. The trend graph is time based and provides a way to relate events to when they occurred. Unfortunately, due to the limited memory of most pacemakers these graphs are limited in their duration. They are programmable to display either heart rate (atrial or ventricular) or sensor rate. In the "rolling" or "final" mode, the events of a past period of time (e.g., 15 minutes) are displayed (Fig. 7.11). This uses the FIFO (first in, first out) algorithm such that only the most recent period of time is available. Earlier data are overwritten as the newest data are obtained. In the "frozen" or "initial" mode, events are recorded until the memory is full. No more data are collected regardless of the time that passes. In some cases the data recorded are not actual event rates, but an average rate of a number of events. Each data point represents the average of 4, 16, 64 or 264 events.

Fig. 7.10. Sensor Indicated Rate Histogram. This type of histogram shows what the sensor activity has been since it was last cleared. It shows what the heart rates would be if the patient was paced 100% of the time. The actual heart rates cannot be determined from this type of plot if the patient's intrinsic heart rate exceeds that of the sensor indicated rate. However, this histogram is still very useful to determine if the sensor is adjusted properly.

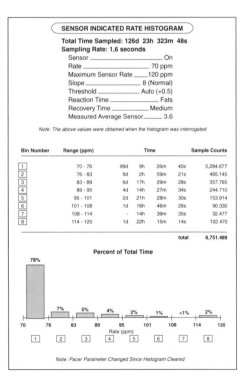

SENSOR INDICATED RATE HISTOGRAM

Total Time Sampled: 126d 23h 323m 48s
Sampling Rate: 1,6 seconds

Sensor _____ On
Rate _____ 70 ppm
Maximum Sensor Rate ____120 ppm
Slope _____ 8 (Normal)
Threshold _____ Auto (+0.5)
Reaction Time _____ Fats
Recovery Time _____ Medium
Measured Average Sensor ____ 3.6

Note: The above values were obtained when the histogram was interrogated

Bin Number	Range (ppm)	Time				Sample Counts
1	70 - 76	99d	9h	26m	40s	5,284.677
2	76 - 83	9d	2h	59m	21s	485.145
3	83 - 89	6d	17h	29m	28s	357.765
4	89 - 95	4d	14h	27m	34s	244.710
5	95 - 101	2d	21h	28m	30s	153.914
6	101 - 108	1d	16h	46m	26s	90.330
7	108 - 114	-	14h	39m	35s	32.477
8	114 - 120	1d	22h	15m	14s	102.470
					total	6,751.489

Percent of Total Time

78%　7%　5%　4%　2%　1%　<1%　2%

70　76　83　89　95　101　108　114　120
Rate (ppm)

1　2　3　4　5　6　7　8

Note: Pacer Parameter Changed Since Histogram Cleared

Some pacemakers now include the ability to trend internal diagnostic features such as lead impedance, R and P-wave amplitudes, and capture thresholds. This is very useful to determine if a problem is developing or has occurred on one of the leads. A progressive drop in the lead impedance would be a clear visual signal that the lead insulation was failing (Fig 7.12).

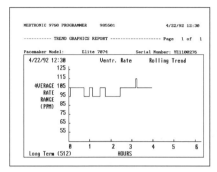

Fig. 7.11. Rolling Trend. This type of plot shows how events occur plotted against time. The frequency of sampling may be from each event, or a number of consecutive events may be averaged to give a single data point in time.

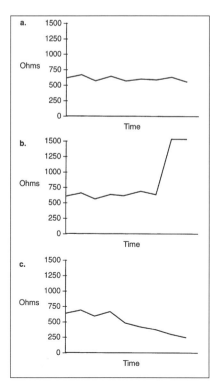

Fig. 7.12. Lead resistance graphs showing (a) normal variation, (b) an abrupt jump in impedance due to a coil fracture, and (c) a gradual decline as is commonly seen with failure of the insulation separating the anode and cathode of a bipolar lead.

Fig. 7.13. The Event Record can be used to "zoom in" to individual heart rhythm events that have occurred over the past several hours. This is an example of a DDD pacemaker. Note the aterisk that corresponds to a PVE (premature ventricular event). The patient was having palpitations which would correlate to these events. The presence of this feature saved having to use a Holter monitor on the patient.

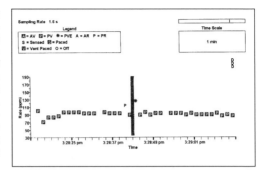

The most advanced method of recording these events currently available is known as the "event record." This can be programmed to sample the heart rate and paced sequence of every beat over a 4 hour period (Fig 7.13). It may also be set to sample less frequently and maintain the data over a longer period. These records present a lot of data and provide a "zoom in" feature on an area that appears suspicious, or during a time when a patient was symptomatic. Some devices allow the patient to place a magnet over the pacemaker when symptoms of palpitations or lightheadedness occur to freeze that portion of the event record in the pacemaker memory. This valuable diagnostic tool, known as a patient triggered event monitor, operates similar to a loop memory event recorder. The saved events can be retrieved and played back on the pacemaker programmer to show what the pacemaker was doing during the symptomatic period. Retrieval of the actual rhythm strip and intracardiac electrogram is not currently available in pacemakers. This added feature will be present in the near future.

Indications for Permanent Pacemaker Implantation

The indications for cardiac pacing have just undergone revision by a joint task force of the American Heart Association and the American College of Cardiology. The most recent revision to the guidelines was published in 1998. As with most procedures the indications for pacing are divided into three broad categories. Class I indications are generally agreed upon and supported by data to be necessary for the patient. Class II indications are those for which there is some disagreement and less data to support implanting a pacemaker. However, pacemakers are frequently implanted for Class II indications. Class II is now subdivided into IIa (weight of evidence/opinion is in favor of usefulness/efficacy) and IIb (usefulness/efficacy is less well established by evidence/opinion). Class III is for situations where pacing is not indicated or not proven to be of any benefit. It is generally considered inappropriate to implant a pacemaker for a Class III situation. The following is a listing by class of indication.

CLASS I: GENERAL AGREEMENT THAT A DEVICE IS INDICATED

Complete heart block, permanent or intermittent, at any anatomic level associated with any one of the following:

- symptomatic bradycardia
- congestive heart fialure
- conditions requiring the use of drugs that suppress escape rates resulting in symptomatic bradycardia
- asystole greater than 3 seconds or escape rate less than 40 bpm without symptoms in awake patients
- confusional states that clear with temporary pacing
- AV-node ablation
- postoperative complete AV-Block that is not expected to resolve
- neuromuscular disorders such as myotonic dystrophy, Kearns-Sayre syndrome, Erbís dystrophy, and peroneal muscular atrophy

Second degree AV-block, permanent or intermittent, regardless of type or site, with symptomatic bradycardia

Handbook of Cardiac Pacing, by Charles J. Love. © 1998 Landes Bioscience

Atrial fibrillation or flutter with complete heart block or advanced AV-block and bradycardia unrelated to digitalis or other drugs (unless needed), with any of the conditions noted for complete AV-block

Persistent advanced 2nd degree AV block (below the AV-node) with bilateral bundle branch block or complete AV-block after acute myocardial infarction

Persistent, symptomatic advanced 2nd or 3rd degree AV block (distal conduction system) after acute myocardial infarction

Transient advanced AV block and associated bilateral bundle branch block postmyocardial infarction

Documented symptomatic sinus bradycardia, possibly due to long term essential drug therapy for which there is no reasonable alternative

Symptomatic chronotropic incompetence (inability to increase heart rate appropriately in response to physiology and/or metabolic demands)

Recurrent syncope with clear spontaneous events provoked by carotid sinus stimulation; minimal carotid sinus pressure causing a pause greater than 3 seconds

Bi- or trifascicular block and intermittent complete or Mobitz-II AV block with or without symptoms

Sustained, pause dependent ventricular tachycardia. The efficacy of pacing must be documented.

CLASS II: DEVICES FREQUENTLY USED, BUT SOME DIVERGENCE OF OPINION WITH RESPECT TO THE NECESSITY OF THEIR INSERTION

CLASS IIA: WEIGHT OF EVIDENCE/OPINION IS IN FAVOR OF USEFULNESS/ EFFICACY

Asymptomatic complete heart block at any anatomic level of the conduction system and ventricular rates of 40 bpm or faster

Asymptomatic Mobitz II block, permanent or intermittent

Asymptomatic Mobitz I at the intra-His or infra-His levels

First degree AV block with symptoms suggestive of pacemaker syndrome, and documented correction of symptoms with temporary AV pacing

Heart rate less than 40 bpm without a clear correlation between symptoms and the bradycardia

Recurrent syncope, but no clear provocative events, and hypersensitive CS response

Syncope of unknown origin with major abnormalities of SA or AV node function documented or provoked during electrophysiologic study.

Bi- or trifascicular block and syncope without proven AV-block, when other causes have been excluded

Bi- or trifascicular block and markedly prolonged HV interval (>100ms)

Bi- or trifascicular block and pacing induced infra-His block

High risk patients with congenital long QT syndrome

CLASS IIB: USEFULNESS/EFFICACY IS LESS WELL ESTABLISHED BY EVIDENCE/ OPINION

> First degree AV block in excess of 300 msec in patients with LV dysfunction and symptoms of CHF, in whom a shorter AV interval results in hemodynamic improvement.
>
> Advanced block at the AV node post myocardial infarction
>
> Minimal symptoms and heart rates less than 30
>
> AV reentrant or AV node reentrant SVT not responsive to medical or ablative therapy
>
> Prevention of symptomatic, drug-refractory, recurrent atrial fibrillation
>
> Recurrent syncope with bradycardia induced by head up tilt testing, the benefit of pacing proven by temporary pacing
>
> Hypertrophic obstructive cardiomyopathy with a significant gradient at rest or provoked

CLASS III: GENERAL AGREEMENT THAT DEVICE IS NOT INDICATED

> Asymptomatic 1st degree AV block
>
> Asymptomatic Mobitz I AV block (above the the bundle of His)
>
> Transient AV block that is expected to resolve and not likely to occur again (e.g. Lyme disease, drug toxicity)
>
> Transient AV block in the absence of an intraventricular conduction delay post myocardial infarction
>
> Transient AV block with isolated left anterior fascicular block post myocardial infarction
>
> Acquired left anterior fascicular block without AV block post myocardial infarction
>
> Persistent 1st degree AV block and bundle branch block that is old or of uncertain age postmyocardial infarction
>
> Bifascicular block but no AV block or symptoms
>
> Bifascicular block and first degree AV block without symptoms
>
> Asymptomatic heart rates less than 40 bpm (possibly due to drug therapy), or when symptoms are clearly not associated with bradycardia
>
> Bradycardia associated with nonessential drug therapy
>
> Hypersensitive carotid sinus response without clinical symptoms
>
> Vague symptoms (dizzy, lightheaded) with hyperactive carotid sinus response
>
> Recurrent syncope, lightheadedness or dizziness in the absence of cardioinhibitory response to tilt table testing.
>
> Vasovagal syncope that is avoidable by behavioral changes
>
> Long QT syndrome due to reversible causes
>
> Frequent or complex ventricular ectopy without sustained VT in the absence of long QT
>
> Patients with hypertrophic obstructive cardiomyopathy who are asymptomatic and/or medically controlled
>
> Hypertrophic cardiomyopathy without evidence of outflow obstruction.

8

ADDITIONAL CONSIDERATIONS

Virtually all of the Class I indications refer to symptoms. It is critical that these be documented in the medical record to show that the pacemaker implant was indicated. It is also very valuable for medical, legal and reimbursement reasons to have in the chart an ECG strip that shows the bradycardia or heart block. Ideally, the correlation between the symptoms and the bradycardia is documented in the medical record. The symptoms that are looked for as being associated with bradycardia are:

Transient dizziness, lightheadedness
Presyncope or syncope
Confusional states
Marked exercise intolerance
Congestive heart failure

Sometimes the indication for pacing may be questionable or fall into a borderline category. For these patients there are other issues that should be considered:

Overall physical and mental state of the patient
Presence of underlying cardiac disease
Patient's desire to operate a motor vehicle
Remoteness from medical care
Necessity of rate depressing drugs
Slowing of basic escape rates
Presence of significant cerebrovascular disease
Desires of patient and family

The presence of a life limiting disease or a patient with irreversible brain damage may not be a suitable candidate for pacing. Patients with severe ischemic disease may require a pacemaker to allow the administration of beta blockers or other drugs that result in symptomatic bradycardia. If a patient lives a great distance from medical care, needs to operate a motor vehicle or has the strong urging of the family, a borderline indication may provide enough of a reason to implant a pacemaker. Conversely, if a patient or the family has strong feelings against an implant then a borderline indication might not provide the physician with enough of a reason to push the issue.

Follow-Up of Permanent Pacemakers

INTRODUCTION

Follow-up of implanted pacemakers is an essential and critical part of patient care. Failure to insure follow-up or to perform it properly may lead to premature battery wear, failure to provide pacing support when needed, and failure to identify problems with the pacemaker before they result in serious consequences for the patient. Ideally, the pacemaker follow-up should be performed by qualified health care personnel that are familiar with both the patient's medical status as well as the device that is implanted. The use of "sales representatives" to perform this function in an unsupervised setting should not be considered acceptable. It is highly desirable for persons involved in pacemaker follow-up to be competent, preferably demonstrated by having taken and passed the NASPE Exam for Competency in Pacing and Defibrillation.

The rationale for regularly scheduled clinic evaluations is as follows:

1. Allow maximum utilization of the pacemaker power source without endangering the patient. This is accomplished by programming the pacemaker to the lowest output that still provides an adequate safety margin allowing for any periodic changes in capture threshold.
2. Detect pacemaker system abnormalities through use of the telemetry features and pacemaker self diagnostic capabilities before symptoms or device failure occur.
3. Permit diagnosis of the nature of device abnormalities before re-operating and allowing correction noninvasively if possible.
4. Allow evaluation and adjustment of sensor-driven pacemakers using histograms and trending graphs to insure that appropriate device response is present between evaluations.
5. Provide an opportunity for continuing patient education regarding their device.
6. Serve as a periodic contact for the patient with the health care system for patients that may otherwise not follow-up with a physician.
7. Provide updated information concerning patient's location and pacemaker related data should there be a recall or alert for the pacemaker or pacing lead.

A simple pacemaker clinic consists of a room with ECG monitoring capability, the appropriate programming equipment, and a pacemaker magnet. More sophisticated centers with dedicated pacemaker services will have a selection of different programmers for many makes and models of devices. They will also have equipment to measure the pulse duration of the pacemaker output and the ability to display a magnified view of the pace artifact. Computer based databases for following the patient and storing ECG data are widely used. This facilitates searches to find a patient with a specific device, or a group of patients when a recall occurs.

PROTOCOL FOR PACEMAKER EVALUATION

There are many methods for evaluating a pacemaker's function. The approach to the patient presenting for a routine evaluation at our institution is as follows:

1. Brief patient history related to heart rhythm symptoms, exertional capability and general cardiovascular status.
2. Examination of the implant site. Additional directed physical examination such as blood pressure determination, chest and cardiac auscultation are performed as indicated.
3. The patient is attached to ECG monitor and the baseline cardiac rhythm is observed for proper device function. A recording is made to document proper or aberrant function. Optionally, a 12 -lead ECG may also be obtained.
4. A magnet is applied over the pacemaker and another recording is made. The magnet rate is calculated and noted.
5. The pacemaker is interrogated and the initial programmed parameters, the measured data, and the diagnostic patient data are printed. These data are evaluated for proper device function and proper response to the patient's needs.
6. While monitored, the patient's intrinsic heart rhythm and level of pacemaker dependence is determined. This is done by reducing the lower pacing rate of the device to see if an intrinsic (nonpaced) rhythm is present. The sensing threshold is evaluated by making the pacemaker less sensitive until it is no longer inhibited by the intrinsic events.
7. If the pacemaker is functioning in the unipolar polarity for sensing, evaluation for myopotential inhibition and/or tracking at the final sensitivity settings is checked for by having the patient do isometric arm exercises while observing the ECG.
8. The capture threshold is determined by reducing the output until capture is lost. Many devices have programmer assisted methods for determining capture. These enhance the safety of the threshold check in patients who do not have an escape rhythm (pacemaker dependent). This feature should be used routinely due to the safety of this method.
9. Based on the threshold determination, the final pacemaker parameters are programmed. For chronic implants in devices without automatic

threshold testing or capture confirmation features, the voltage is programmed at 1.7 to 2 times the threshold value measured at a pulse width of .3 to .6 msec. Alternatively, if the threshold was measured by keeping the voltage stable and reducing the pulse width, the pulse width may be tripled. The latter method is valid only if the pulse width threshold is .3 msec or less.

10. The patient is provided with a printout of the final parameters, informing them of the demand rate and upper rate limit (if applicable). By allowing the patient to keep a copy of the programmed parameters they are able to present it to health care personnel in the emergency room or at other institutions. This can save many phone calls to the pacemaker clinic or the physician who is on call.

11. A chest X-ray may be taken at routine intervals (e.g., yearly) at the discretion of the physician.

Adjustments to the device and the frequency of device evaluation should be made with consideration of the level of risk to the individual patient. Factors to consider are listed in Table 9.1.

Transtelephonic follow-up is a means by which the pacemaker clinic is able to obtain a rhythm strip over the phone. The capability to reprogram the pacemaker over the telephone is not currently available. With newer and more advanced transmitters we have just begun to have the capability to receive diagnostic data and telemetry information from the pacemakers. However, the current standard methodology for telephone evaluation has not changed in two decades. It provides for the transmission of a real time rhythm strip by having the patient place a small device on the chest or by using a set of metal bracelets attached to the transmitter (Fig 9.1). This device generates a tone that is decoded into a rhythm strip by a receiving center (Fig 9.2). This is useful in conjunction with magnet application to determine if the pacemaker is functioning and to get a general idea as to the condition of the battery. It does not replace the full evaluation that is performed in the pacemaker clinic. An additional benefit of these transmitters is that the patient can send a rhythm strip during an episode of palpitations.

The rationale for routine transtelephonic follow-up is as follows:

1. Makes available a method for monitoring the continued safety and longevity of the pacing system between office visits.

Table 9.1. Risk considerations for programming and follow-up frequency

Degree of pacemaker dependency
Device advisories or recalls on the pacemaker or leads
Changes in underlying heart disease
Severity of underlying heart disease
Epicardial electrodes
Pediatric patients
Exposure to cardioversion, defibrillation, or electrocautery
High stimulation thresholds with high programmed outputs
Undersensing, interference or other sensing problems
Concurrent use of an ICD or other implanted device

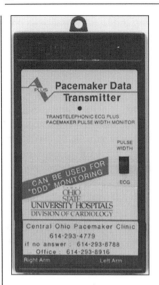 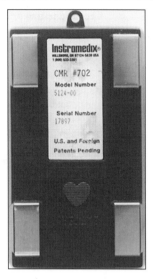

Fig. 9.1a and b. Front and back of basic transmitter. The four metal feet are dampened with water and applied to the chest. The mouthpiece of the telephone is held over the front of the transmitter to send an analog signal to the receiving center.

Fig. 9.1c. Cradle type transmitter packaged with a magnet. The phone is placed in the cradle and the wrist bands are placed on the patient to acquire the electrocardiogram.

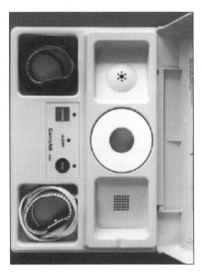

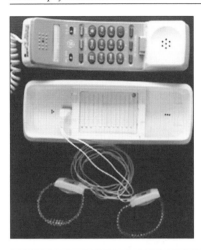

Fig. 9.1d. Cardiophone™ Transmitter integrated into a standard telephone set. The patient may use the phone for routine calls, and plug in the wrist bands to transmit to the pacing center when needed.

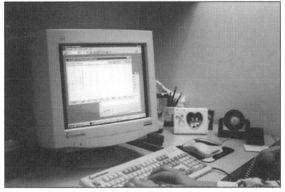

Fig. 9.2. Typical transtelephonic receiving center. This Paceart™ system is computer based and runs on a standard "PC". Analysis, reporting and storage of the transmitted rhythm strip is performed efficiently as opposed to the "cut and paste" method of the older style heated pen strip recorders.

9

2. Provides a method of detecting pacemaker system abnormalities before symptoms occur.
3. Allows transmission of a rhythm strip into the clinic office when patient is symptomatic.
4. For patients that are not able to come to the pacemaker clinic, this provides at least a minimal level of follow-up.

The standard procedure for routine transtelephonic evaluation at most centers is as follows:

1. The patient is questioned as to their general health status as well as any symptoms that relate to cardiac rhythm.
2. Transmission of the rhythm for 30 seconds without a magnet.
3. Transmission of the rhythm for 30 seconds with a magnet over the pacemaker.
4. The magnet is removed and another 30 seconds of rhythm is recorded.

5. The patient is assured that the pacemaker function is normal. If a problem is found the patient has the situation explained. Arrangement is made for a more thorough evaluation in the clinic or for corrective action to be taken as indicated.

There is some concern that pacing a patient asynchronously could provoke a ventricular or atrial arrhythmia. This could occur by delivering a pace output during the vulnerable period of the cardiac cycle (R on T). While this is theoretically possible, it occurs extremely infrequently in clinical practice. For any patient that has demonstrated a predisposition towards significant arrhythmia from magnet application, this type of testing should be avoided unless done in a proper medically supervised environment.

FREQUENCY OF FOLLOW-UP

There are two approaches for routine evaluation in the clinic and by telephone; Medicare guidelines and the NASPE guidelines. The former were developed for pacemakers that are no longer in general use. They are antiquated and are used by those who, in general, wish to maximize clinic revenue. The latter are more rational and were developed with regard to the modern pacemakers. We use the NASPE guidelines and strongly encourage others to do so as well. Follow-up frequency should be adjusted based on the patient's needs. These may be more frequent if medically justified. The Medicare and NASPE guidelines are presented below.

MEDICARE GUIDELINES FOR PACEMAKER FOLLOW-UP

Pacemaker Clinic Monitoring:
    Single chamber pacemakers
        Twice the first 6 months following implant
        Once every 12 months.
    Dual chamber pacemakers:
        Twice the first 6 months following implant
        Once every 6 months.
Transtelephonic Monitoring (TTM):Guideline 1**
    Single chamber pacemakers
        1st month q 2 weeks
        2nd–36th months q 8 weeks
        37th and later q 4 weeks
    Dual chamber pacemakers
        1st month q 2 weeks
        2nd–6th months q 4 weeks
        7th–36th months q 8 weeks
        36th month and later q 4 weeks

9

Transtelephonic Monitoring (TTM):Guideline 2**

> Single chamber pacemakers
>> 1st month q 2 weeks
>> 2nd–48th months q 12 weeks
>> 49th–72nd month q 8 weeks
>> 73rd month and later q 4 weeks
>
> Dual chamber pacemakers
>> 1st month q 2 weeks
>> 2nd–30th months q 12 weeks
>> 31st–48th month q 8 weeks
>> 49th month and later q 4 weeks

**Medicare guideline 2 is for pacemakers that have demonstrated better than 90% longevity at 5 years, whose output voltage decreases less than 50% over at least 3 months and whose magnet rate decreases less than 20% or 5 pulses per minute over the same period. Virtually all modern pacemakers would fall under this guideline.

Guideline 1 is for devices that do not meet the above criteria.

NASPE GUIDELINES FOR PACEMAKER FOLLOW-UP

9

Predischarge:
> Full clinic evaluation + PA & Lateral CXR and 12-lead ECG, Provide TTM transmitter and training in its use.

1st Outpatient Follow-up (6-8 weeks postimplant)
> Full clinic evaluation
> Programming changes to chronic values
> Review patient education and retention of concepts
> TTM only as required for symptoms prior to this visit

Early Surveillance Period (through 5th month)
> One clinic or one TTM contact

Maintenance Period (beginning at 6 months)
> Full Clinic evaluation yearly.
> TTM with patient interview q3 months, unless clinic evaluation is performed near scheduled TTM.

Intensified Period (Latest interval in the Medicare schedule or when battery shows significant wear)
> Full Clinic evaluation yearly
> TTM with patient interview q1 month, unless clinic evaluation is performed near a scheduled TTM.

For older pacemakers that are not showing significant signs of battery wear there is really no need to perform monthly TTM evaluations unless indicated for other reasons such as device reliability or recalls.

Preoperative, Operative and Postoperative Considerations

PREOPERATIVE PREPARATION OF THE PATIENT

Education of the patient is critical to ensure that there are appropriate expectations regarding both the operative procedure as well as the outcome. It is important that the patient understand not only what the pacemaker will do, but what it will not do. Patients expecting that their gout will be cured or that their aortic valve stenosis will resolve with a pacemaker implant will be quite disappointed. Patients with appropriate expectations will be very satisfied. It is important to give an adequate explanation to reduce the apprehension and anxiety that is normal. Important points to cover during the explanation include:

1. The indication for pacing
2. An explanation of the type of pacemaker chosen
3. A description of the basic function of the pacemaker
4. Determination of the site of the incision. This should be done with consideration as to dominant hand, prior chest or breast surgery, chest or clavicular injury, known vascular anomaly and special sporting or other needs.
5. The type of sedation, analgesia and anesthesia to be used
6. A general description of the surgical technique
7. The risks of the operation

Prior to the operation, routine orders may include some or all of the following:

1. NPO for 6-8 hours
2. Basic laboratory studies (CBC, differential, electrolytes, BUN, creatinine, PT, PTT, platelet count)
3. Discontinuation of anticoagulants and aspirin if possible
4. 18 ga or larger intravenous access
5. Shave insertion area
6. Antiseptic soap bath or shower to area where incision is to be made
7. Void bladder on call to the operating room

8. Prophylactic antibiotic (e.g., vancomycin, cefazolin, etc.)
9. Analgesia/sedation (e.g., midazolam, meperidine, etc.)

PACEMAKER POCKET LOCATION

As noted above, the location for the site of the pacemaker implant in the body should be based on the patient needs and not on physician convenience. It is preferred that the nondominant side be used to minimize the exposure to flexion of the implanted lead as it passes under the clavicle. Most patients find that having the pacemaker on the dominant side is less comfortable and that it seems to "get in the way." If the patient has had a mastectomy then the opposite side should be used as more tissue will be present to cover the pacemaker. Patients that like to hunt may use either shoulder to brace the weapon. They should be asked which shoulder they use for shooting so the device may be placed on the opposite side. It is not considered good medical practice to have a gun lover angry at the physician. A history of clavicular fracture or edema of an upper extremity should alert one to the possibility of anatomic or vascular abnormalities that could make the implant a challenge. Golfers present a true challenge as no matter which side one places the device they will claim you ruined their game. In some cases the upper chest is not appropriate for implant, or the transvenous route is not available from above. In this case the pacemaker may be placed in the abdominal wall. Epicardial leads are placed on the heart or alternate venous approaches may be considered. For most pacemakers, the pocket is made in the prepectoral region, one or two centimeters below and parallel to the clavicle. If the cephalic vein is used the incision may be in the deltopectoral groove.

10

LEAD INSERTION

The venous system is usually accessed for lead placement using a subclavian vein cannulation or cephalic vein cutdown. The cutdown technique virtually eliminates the risk of pneumothorax or hemothorax. It does take a bit more time to perform, and occasionally only a small vein is found. Both approaches are common, however when diagnosing postoperative complications it is useful to know which was used. On rare occasions the internal jugular vein may be used and the lead tunneled over or under the clavicle to the pocket area.

LEAD POSITIONING

Transvenous ventricular leads have been typically placed in the right ventricular apex, and transvenous atrial leads in the right atrial appendage. However, leads may be placed in other positions as well. The use of active fixation leads with a helix to screw them into the myocardium allows stable positioning in virtually any position. New data suggests that ventricular leads placed high on the intraventricular septum or in the right ventricular outflow tract will improve stroke volume as compared to lead placement in the apex. This may be due to a more synchronized depolarization with the left ventricle. Atrial leads may be placed anywhere in the right atrium as long as the thresholds for sensing and pacing are good. If a lateral position for the atrial lead is used it is essential to be sure that the phrenic nerve does not get stimulated with atrial pacing. Epicardial leads may be screwed in, stabbed in, or sutured on. The approach to placing them on the heart may be via sternotomy, thoracotomy (limited or otherwise) or subxyphoid.

Congenital anomalies may make transvenous lead placement difficult or impossible. The most common anomaly is the "persistent left superior vena cava". In this situation the left inominate vein does not cross over to meet the right inominate to form the superior vena cava. Instead, the left inominate stays on the left side of the chest and empties into the coronary sinus via the great cardiac vein. This anomaly occurs in approximately 1% of the population. Though more difficult to place, both single and dual chamber pacing systems may be inserted via this route. Obviously, if the presence of this anomaly is known ahead of time the implant would be best done on the right side. Other less common anomalies are related to repairs of congenital defects such as transposition of the great vessels. Issues regarding these problems are beyond the scope of this publication. One must be aware that they exist as the X-ray appearance may be unusual.

COMPLICATIONS OF PACEMAKER INSERTION

As with any surgical procedure there are many potential complications. Many of these may be avoided by careful planning and performance of the procedure. However, even in the best and most experienced hands problems may arise. It is vital that a problem be identified as soon as possible so that corrective action may be initiated. I have divided the types of complications into three categories as shown in Table 10.1. Most of the listed problems are self explanatory. The "Twiddler" syndrome is caused by a patient (often with Alzheimer's Disease) flipping the pacemaker over and over in the pocket. This causes the lead to wind up much like a telephone cord that twists over on itself. The lead may be pulled out of the heart by tension or the lead may be damaged by the severe stress caused by torsion.

PACEMAKER LEAD EXTRACTION

When a pacing lead becomes infected or when certain other complications arise it may be necessary to remove a chronically implanted lead or group of leads. If the lead has been implanted less than one year, it will likely (but not always) pull out of the heart with minimal traction. Leads that have been implanted for more than a year begin to aggressively fibrose to the vascular and myocardial tissues. Over time they become encased in scar tissue and even calcified. This makes them difficult and potentially dangerous to remove. The indications based on a scheme

Table 10.1. Complications of pacemaker insertion

Lead Insertion Related:
   Pneumothorax
   Hemothorax
   Subclavian artery injury
   Air embolus
   Thoracic duct injury
   Brachial plexus injury
   Chordae or valve entanglement/rupture
   Tricuspid insufficiency by the lead holding the valve open
   Cardiac perforation
   Pericardial tamponade
Lead Related (other):
   Diaphragm pacing (chest wall or phrenic nerve)
   Endocarditis
   Insulation failure/damage
   Lead conductor failure
   Lead connector failure
   Lead dislodgment
   Exit block (high-capture threshold)
   Loss of sensing
   Venous thrombosis
   Poor connection at generator
   Malposition in the coronary sinus
   Malposition across a patent foramen ovale or atrial septal defect
Pocket Related:
   Hematoma
   Erosion
   Infection
   Chronic pain
   Migration of pacemaker
   "Twiddler" syndrome
   Pectoralis muscle stimulation
   Pocket stimulation

10

published by Charles Byrd for removal of chronically implanted pacing leads are listed in Table 10.2. The indications are currently under review and will be published by NASPE in the near future. Mandatory reasons for removing a pacing lead are the result of a condition that is or could be life threatening, while necessary reasons are to correct a problem. Some problems do not cause an immediate medical threat, but one might wish to prevent future problems. In some cases it is simply to the patient's advantage to have the leads removed. These latter two situations fall under the discretionary category.

Leads, pacemakers and defibrillators that are infected present a difficult therapeutic problem. An infection involving only the incision and not the implanted hardware may be curable with antibiotics. If the pocket itself is infected or if a portion of the lead, pacemaker or defibrillator has eroded, antibiotics are unlikely to result in a cure. At best, suppression of the infection will be possible until the antibiotics are stopped. All of the prosthetic material must be removed from the

---

Table 10.2. Indications for extraction of pacing leads

Mandatory
    Endocarditis
    Sepsis due to the pacing system
    Obliteration of all usable veins
    Mishap during attempted extraction
    Traumatic injury to the lead / vein site
Necessary
    Pocket infection
    Occult infection
    Erosion of the pacemaker or lead
    Chronic draining sinus
    Multiple leads in a single vessel
Discretionary
    Malignancy
    Pocket pain
    Deteriorating polyurethane insulation
    Accufix and Encor "J" leads*

---

*The need for removal of these leads will depend on the individual patient and the risk benefit ratio as determined by the physician. The actual classification for extraction of these leads will depend on the clinical situation. Elderly patients with normal leads need not have them removed. Younger patients ought to have the leads extracted as a precautionary measure. Patients with failed leads and protruding wires should have the leads removed under most circumstances. Consultation with a lead extraction expert is recommended in situations involving this lead.

10

patient to insure a cure. Infected pockets must be excised or left open to heal by secondary intention. Patients with sepsis or endocarditis caused by the pacing system must be treated aggressively with antibiotics and removal of all hardware.

Removal of pacing leads used to require an open heart procedure when they would not come out with traction. Eventually, the "weight and pulley" method was used. This technique was performed by exposing the pacing lead and tying a piece of suture to it. The suture was then run over a pulley and a small weight was tied to it. The patient was placed on a nursing unit until the weight crashed to the floor. It was at this time that all would know that the lead had pulled free from the heart. While this was a somewhat effective (not to mention dramatic) method of removing leads, it was time consuming and the same implant site could not be reused as it had been exposed for too long a period of time. Over the past decade the use of locking stylets and counter traction sheaths have been developed to provide a safe and rapid method to consistently remove leads. The locking stylets stabalize the lead and provide traction at the tip of the lead. The sheaths are passed over the lead to tear away adhesive scar tissue, and to provide a localized force at the lead myocardial interface to prevent an avulsion. More recently the Excimer laser has been approved for use in the removal of pacing leads. It is used to vaporize the scar tissue instead of tearing it away. The laser energy is delivered by a fiberoptic sheath that is passed over the lead. When the sheath encounters a binding site energy is applied and the sheath vaporizes the tissue. Though highly effective, this is an expensive methodology. Lead extraction is a difficult and potentially dangerous procedure. It should only be performed by physicians well trained and experienced in the technique, and at centers that are capable of dealing with the potential life threatening problems that can occur.

POSTOPERATIVE MANAGEMENT OF THE PACEMAKER PATIENT

Postoperative management of the patient is directed at insuring that the device is functioning properly and at minimizing pain and the risk of wound problems. Common postoperative orders are listed in Table 10.3.

Many physicians obtain not only the PA and lateral chest X-ray on the following day, but also a STAT portable film to rule out a pneumothorax. We obtain this extra film only if there is a suspicion that the pleura was penetrated or if the patient becomes symptomatic. The ice pack to the site helps to reduce edema and pain. The use of IV antibiotics is always controversial. Most surgical literature supports the use of a single dose preoperatively as prophylaxis against infection. The use of additional antibiotic postoperatively is not proven to reduce the incidence of infection. However, most implanting physicians give at least one additional dose. Maintaining the head of the bed slightly elevated will help to keep the venous pressures in the upper body lower and reduce the amount of bleeding into the pacemaker pocket. Some physicians restrict the movement of the patient's arm with a sling to reduce the risk of lead dislodgment in the early postoperative period. We have found that if the leads are properly secured and are placed with the right amount of slack that dislodgment is very unlikely with or without the sling. Indeed, if a lead is going to dislodge it tends to do so when the PA X-ray is taken. It is during this time that the patient is standing with arms raised over the X-ray plate during a deep inspiration. I have found this to be the ultimate test of lead stability.

The pacemaker should be thoroughly evaluated prior to patient discharge. This includes threshold checks, sensor evaluation and adjustment, activation of special features and counters, and a final interrogation with printing of all programmed parameters. The patient will have many questions that will require answers. In addition, final instructions regarding wound care and follow-up must be discussed. A summary of the instructions that we give our patients is presented in Table 10.4.

Most of the issues listed in Table 10.4 are straightforward. However, issues involving electromagnetic interference (EMI) are of concern to both patients and physicians. If the pacemaker does sense EMI, it will usually recognize this as abnormal and nonphysiologic. As the EMI will "blind" the pacemaker to the patient's heart rhythm, it will begin to pace asynchronously at an "interference rate." This is usually around 60 or 70 bpm. It does this to be sure that the patient is not without pacing support during this time. The patient may notice a change in the heart rhythm due to loss of AV synchrony or competition with the native rhythm. The pacemaker will resume normal function when the source is turned off or if the patient moves away from it.

10

Table 10.3. Common postoperative orders

1. PA and Lateral chest X-ray within 2 hrs for lead placement and to evaluate for pneumothorax
2. Ice pack to incision site
3. IV antibiotics (usually one additional dose)
4. Oral and parenteral analgesics
5. Maintain head of bead > 30° angle
6. Resumption of diet
7. Vital signs frequently at first then tapering to routine
8. Wound dressing check for drainage and hematoma
9. Respiratory status evaluation (for pneumothorax)
10. Monitor ECG rhythm for arrhythmias, capture and appropriate sensing
11. Restrict movement of ipsilateral arm for 24 hours
12. Full pacemaker evaluation prior to discharge with activation of any special features and adjustment of the sensor if present

Table 10.4. Predischarge teaching

Wound care instructions include the following:
1. Continually assess wound for signs and symptoms of infection.
2. Keep wound clean and dry for 1 week.
3. Cover the incision with plastic when bathing.
4. Remove steri-strips after 7 days. Do not wait until they fall off.

Activity restrictions:
1. No lifting greater than 10 pounds for 2 weeks.
2. No repetitive arm extension over the head for 2 weeks.
3. If the patient is pacemaker dependent, driving should be restricted for 2 weeks or as determined by the physician. Otherwise, 48 hours is usually sufficient to allow the patient to recover from any anesthesia and for the incisional pain to subside

Restrictions against electromagnetic interference:
1. Arc welding
2. MRI
3. Diathermy
4. Therapeutic radiation over the pacemaker
5. Electronic article surveillance scanners
6. Metal detectors
7. Supermarket checkout scanners
8. Cell phones
9. Electric blankets

Contact the pacemaker clinic if:
1. Symptoms prior to implant return
2. The pulse rate seems too slow or too fast
3. Dizziness, lightheadedness, or syncope occurs
4. Unusual shortness of breath or chest pain develops
5. Muscle twitching around the pacemaker is present

Virtually all household electrical items and power tools are safe for patients to use. Sources of high electrical energy, such as arc welders, power generators, large electromagnets and the high voltage ignition system of a gasoline engine, may create enough EMI to affect pacemaker function. MRI scanners are a problem for pacemakers due to the high energy radiofrequency energy fields that they generate. They are not likely to suck the pacemaker and wires through the chest as there is very little ferrous metal in these devices other that the reed switch. Metal detectors and article surveillance systems are a problem only if the pacemaker is held directly against the scanner. Metal detectors may be triggered at airports by an implanted device. Showing the security personnel the identification card is usually sufficient to satisfy them that the patient is not a terrorist; however, a hand search may be conducted to be sure. Electric blankets may occasionally cause enough EMI to cause the pacemaker to revert to the interference mode, though this is relatively uncommon.

Finally, the issue of cell phones is constantly raised. The portable phones that are used in the home present no problem to a pacemaker. Cell phones may affect some models of pacemakers. There is significant variability between manufacturers as to the resistance to EMI from these phones. In addition, the newer digital phones that have been used in Europe and are now being introduced into the United States are more likely to cause inhibition of a pacemaker than the analog phones currently in use. Studies have shown that if the phone's antenna is 6 inches or more away from the pacemaker that it is very unlikely to affect the operation of the pacemaker. When patients have a hand held cellular phone we recommend that it be held to the ear opposite the site of the pacemaker implant. It is just as important that the phone not be placed in a pocket over the pacemaker while the phone power is on. This is because a cellular phone is in constant contact with the local transmitters even if it is not "off the hook".

General instructions regarding the patients disease and symptoms are also reviewed prior to discharge. The indications for the pacemaker implant and basics of pacemaker function are reviewed. Most patients have several common questions that will need to be answered. These include:

1. Can I cook with a microwave?
2. What about using household appliances and tools?
3. How long will my pacemaker last?
4. When can I drive?
5. How will I know if my pacemaker malfunctions?
6. What about airport security checks?
7. What happens to my pacemaker when I die?

Most of these questions have been addressed in the preceding section. We tell patients that the microwave oven will only harm the pacemaker if the pacemaker is placed into the oven. Since most patients will not fit in a microwave oven the pacemaker is unlikely to be affected. Older pacemakers were not encased in metal (which reflects microwaves), and older ovens were not sealed as well as the newer ones. It is therefore very uncommon to have a pacemaker affected by this common appliance, even though restaurants and many snack areas in hospitals still display a large sign warning pacemaker patients about the presence of the micro-wave oven. Most modern pacemakers will last in the range of five to ten years. We tell our patients this and explain that it will depend on how the pacemaker is finally programmed and how often they are paced. Obviously a pacemaker that is inhibited 90% of the time will last longer than one that paces 90% of the time. Some patients and family members have concerns about the pacemaker continuing to operate after death has occurred. The thought of the person being dead yet the pacemaker continuing to make the heart beat is a chilling thought. The fact is that the pacemaker will continue to deliver an impulse to the heart but no con-traction will occur as the muscle ceases to function. We get an occasional urgent call from monitored units to turn off the pacemaker because a patient has ex-pired. We ask them to turn off their ECG monitor if the pacemaker spikes bother them. In rare cases a patient may be near death with the pacemaker simply pro-longing the imminent event. The family and physician may then decide that turn-ing off the pacemaker is appropriate.

Prior to discharge a temporary pacemaker identification card that is present in the registration material is given to the patient. This includes the model, serial number and dates of implant for the pacemaker and lead(s). It also has the name of the following physician and a contact phone number. A copy of the programmed parameters is given as a reference for the patient. It is also useful for health care professionals should the patient require medical care elsewhere. It is essential that the pacemaker and leads be registered with their manufacturers. This assists other physicians in identifying the device and allows the company to track the device should there be a recall or alert. Registration is also mandated by Federal law through the Safe Medical Devices Act of 1990.

Evaluation of Pacemaker Malfunction

EVALUATION OF PACEMAKER MALFUNCTION

The first step in evaluating pacemaker malfunction is to determine if the function of the device is truly abnormal or if one is seeing normal function of the device. By far the largest number of consults we see for malfunctioning pacemakers are for devices that are functioning properly. With the advent of so many "special features," it is easy for even a person experienced with pacemakers to misinterpret the normal operation of a pacemaker. Before one spends a great deal of time attempting to troubleshoot a pacemaker it is imperative that the normal function of the pacemaker be understood. This is accomplished by obtaining some basic information about the patient, the device implanted and the programmed parameters (Table 11.1). Many patients carry an identification card that has the information related to the implanted devices. Patients occasionally lose their card or do not bring it with them. As a secondary method to identify the device a chest X-ray may be taken. Pacemakers have a logo, code or distinct radiographic "skeleton" that may be matched to a reference text (Fig. 11.1). If the manufacturer can be identified, a call to the manufacturer's patient registration department can provide the basic information needed. Table 11.2 provides phone numbers in the United States for some of the pacemaker companies.

As with any medical problem, the history is usually the key to determining the cause of a problem or at least to significantly narrowing the diagnostic options. If the problem occurs shortly after implant then lead dislodgment, insufficiently tightened set screws, or poor lead placement should be suspected as a cause rather than battery depletion or lead fracture. Conversely, an older device is more likely to be compromised by lead failure and battery depletion rather than lead dislodgment.

The presence or absence of symptoms is very important. This will determine if urgent action is required or if the luxury of a more leisurely approach to problem solving is appropriate. The first step in a grossly symptomatic patient is to establish a stable cardiac rhythm. If the patient is severely bradycardic and the pacemaker programmer is not available or programming changes to the device are ineffective, temporary transvenous pacing should be established as soon as possible.

11

Handbook of Cardiac Pacing, by Charles J. Love. © 1998 Landes Bioscience

Table 11.1. Basic troubleshooting data requirements

Pacemaker model
Pacemaker serial number
Lead model(s)
Lead serial numbers(s)
Date of implant for each component
Current programming
Measured data
Lead impedance(s)
Battery voltage and / or impedance
Indication for pacing
Chest X-Ray (if needed or indicated)

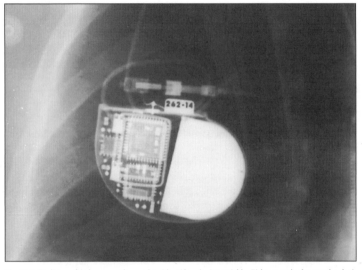

Fig. 11.1. Radiographic logos can be used to identify a device quickly. Either a code that can be deci-
phered by using a book or calling a manufacturer, or a model number may be present. In this radiograph the model number 262-14 is clearly seen, instantly identifying the pacemaker.

If necessary, external pacing may be used until a more definitive solution is a-
vailable.

A tachycardia driven by the pacemaker presents a more difficult situation. In
most cases application of a magnet or a programming change will terminate the
rapid rhythm. In rare cases the pacemaker will not respond and urgent surgical
intervention may be required for "runaway pacemaker" (Fig. 11.2). This uncommon malfunction is caused by a major component failure in the pacing circuit.
The vast majority of rapid pacing rates are caused by a DDD or VDD device tracking

Table 11.2. Phone numbers for pacemaker and ICD manufacturers

Biotronic	800-547-0394
Cardiac Control Systems (CCS)	800-227-7223
Cardiac Pacemakers, Inc (CPI)	800-227-3422
Cordis	800-777-2237
Ela	800-352-6466
In Control	425-861-9301
Medtronic	800-328-2518
Sulzer-Intermedics	888-432-7801
Pacesetter, St. Jude	800-777-2237
Telectronics	800-777-2237
Ventritex	800-777-2237
Vitatron	800-848-2876

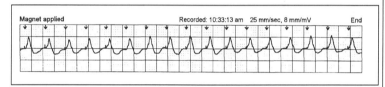

Fig. 11.2. Runaway pacemaker. This strip shows VVI pacing at 180 bpm (the runaway protect limit on this device). The pacemaker was programmed to the DDD mode with an upper rate limit of 120 bpm. Therapeutic radiation delivered to the pacemaker in a pateint with breast cancer resulted in circuit failure and rapid pacing. Even magnet application did not slow the pacing rate. The device was replaced emergently.

11

atrial fibrillation or flutter. The pacemaker will try to track the rapid atrial rate to the upper rate limit of the pacemaker. Placing a magnet over the device will drop the pacing rate to the magnet rate of the device until it can be programmed to a nontracking mode such as DDI or VVI. Sensor-driven devices may cause rapid pacing as well. In one case we found a patient who was experiencing a wide complex tachycardia and a tonic-clonic seizure. The wide complex tachycardia was the result of a vibration based sensor-driven pacemaker responding to the seizure. Note that it is still quite possible for a patient with an intact AV node to have an atrial arrhythmia with rapid ventricular response. Unfortunately the pacemaker is of little help in this situation. Many times the patient and others expect that we will be able to reduce the intrinsic heart rate by reprogramming of the device. This is not true and represents a misunderstanding of the function of a pacemaker.

After the condition of the patient is stabilized, the history obtained, and the initial data concerning the device is obtained, the ECG is evaluated. An approach to determining the general function of the pacing system is detailed in Table 11.3.

Table 11.3. Approach to the ECG

1. Pacing
    a. Spike present
        1) Verify appropriate rate interval
        2) Verify appropriate depolarization response
            a) capture
            b) pseudofusion
            c) fusion
    b. Spike absent
        1) Apply magnet (magnet function must be enabled)
        (Note: a ventricular pacemaker spike falling in the absolute refractory period of
        the myocardium will NOT result in capture.)
        2) Observe on 12 lead ECG for pace artifact and capture.
2. Sensing
    a. Patient must have periods of nonpaced rhythm
    b. Appropriate escape interval—Hysteresis
3. Compare function to known technical information, observing for end of service
    indications and other variations.

Absence of a pacing output may be caused not only by output problems but also by oversensing. An easy way to remember this is that "oversensing causes underpacing, and undersensing causes overpacing." If the pacemaker is sensing an electrical event, the pacemaker will be inhibited. Often times this is a premature ectopic beat that may be isoelectric on a single monitor lead. For this reason multi-lead recordings are needed to evaluate the system properly. Oversensing can be diagnosed quickly by placing a magnet over the device. If pacing resumes while the magnet is in place then oversensing is a problem. If there is no pacing with the magnet on, then either the pacemaker is not putting out a pulse or the pulse is not reaching the heart.

Once the nature of the problem is identified, consideration of the possible causes is necessary so that appropriate corrective action may take place. It must also be understood that a failing pacemaker may manifest any of the following malfunctions due to the unpredictable nature of circuit failure or the effects of low battery voltage on the circuit. Causes of true pacemaker failure are noted in Table 11.4.

NONCAPTURE

This potentially life threatening problem is identified by the presence of pacemaker pulse artifact without capture (QRS or P wave) following the impulse (Fig. 11.3). Causes of noncapture are listed in Table 11.5.

Corrective Action

Increase pacemaker output if possible. Where appropriate, revise or replace lead or pacemaker, correct metabolic imbalances. For pseudo-noncapture adjust the sensitivity to a more sensitive setting.

Table 11.4. Causes of pacemaker failure

Battery depletion
Defibrillation near or over the device
Use of electrocautery near or on the device
Random component failure
Severe direct trauma to the device
Therapeutic radiation directed at or near the device
Known modes of failure for devices on recall or alert

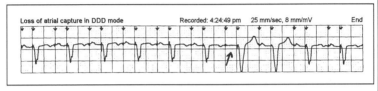

Fig. 11.3a. Atrial noncapture. In this dual chamber device, atrial capture is lost as can be seen by the absence of a P wave, and the sudden appearance of a wide complex QRS.

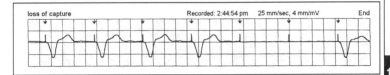

Fig. 11.3b. Ventricular noncapture. Paced output occurs without depolarizing the ventricle resulting in an asystolic pause. This pacemaker was programmed to VVI at 70 bpm.

Table 11.5. Common causes of noncapture

Exit block (high-capture threshold)
Inappropriate programming to a low output or pulse width
Lead dislodgment
Lead fracture
Lead insulation failure
Loose connection to pacemaker
Low battery output
Severe metabolic imbalance
Drug effect
"Pseudo-noncapture" (pacing during the refractory period due to undersensing of the preceding complex)

UNDERSENSING

Recognized by the presence of pulse artifact occurring after an intrinsic event which occurs but does not reset the escape interval (Fig.11.4). This may or may not capture depending on where in the cardiac cycle the pace output falls. Causes of undersensing (thus "overpacing") are listed in Table 11.6.

Corrective Action

Increase pacemaker sensitivity. Where appropriate, revise or replace the lead. If the problem is very infrequent then careful observation may be acceptable.

OVERSENSING

Recognized by inappropriate inhibition of the pacemaker in a single chamber system (Fig.11.5). This may be seen as total inhibition of output or as prolongation of the escape interval. Myopotentials cause a form of oversensing seen

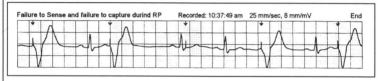

Fig. 11.4. Undersensing. This pacemaker is not sensing any of the intrinsic complexes (pacing asynchronously). The device is programmed to VVI at 45 bpm with a very low sensitivity setting. Note that the 3rd paced output fails to capture as it occurs during the refractory period of the ventricle.

Table 11.6. Causes of undersensing

Poor lead position with poor R-wave or P-wave amplitude
Lead dislodgment
Lead fracture
Lead insulation failure
Severe metabolic disturbance
Defibrillation near pacemaker
Myocardial infarction of tissue near electrode
Ectopic beats of poor intracardiac amplitude
DVI-committed function
Safety pacing

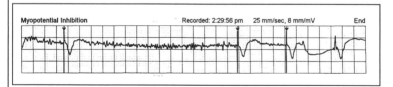

Fig. 11.5. Myopotential inhibition. As the patient begins to use the arm on the same side of the pacemaker, the electrical signals of the pectoralis are sensed and mistaken to be QRS signals. The device is inhibited until the patient relaxes. Note the muscle artifact on the baseline of this rhythm strip.

predominantly in unipolar pacemakers. Inhibition is usually caused by sensing noncardiac muscle activity. Myopotentials are typically caused by arm movements or lifting for prepectoral implants, and by sitting up for abdominal implants. Inhibition may also be caused by the ventricular lead sensing the T-wave. This "fools" the device into believing a cardiac event has occurred. Output is therefore inhibited as long as these signals continue. Dual chamber systems may exhibit tracking of electrical signals such as myopotentials. This is caused by the same mechanisms as is inhibition as just discussed (inhibition may occur in either the atrium, ventricle or both with a dual chamber pacemaker). However, rapid pacing may be the result of oversensing of electrical signals on the atrial channel that are not strong enough to be sensed on (and thus inhibit) the ventricular channel. The atrial channel is usually set to a more sensitive value than the ventricular one. What happens is that an AVI is started each time oversensing occurs triggering a ventricular output at a rate up to the programmed URL. This is demonstrated by tracking of myopotentials on a unipolar system as shown in Figure 11.6. Additional causes of oversensing are listed in Table 11.7.

Corrective Action

Decrease the sensitivity of the device. For far-field or T-wave sensing, prolongation of the refractory period will correct the problem. The sensing polarity may

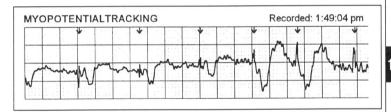

Fig. 11.6. Myopotential tracking. This pacemaker is tracking the patient's sinus rhythm. As the patient begins to use the arm on the same side of the pacemaker, the atrial channel of the pacemaker senses the electrical impulses generated by the pectoralis muscle. The pacemaker "tracks" the myopotentials instead of the P-waves resulting in loss of AV synchrony and rapid ventricular pacing. If the myopotentials inhibit the ventricular channel, asystole may result.

Table 11.7. Causes of oversensing

Myopotentials
Electromagnetic interference
T-wave sensing
Far-field R-wave sensing (atrial lead)
Lead insulation failure
Lead fracture
Loose fixation screw
Crosstalk

---

be reprogrammed to bipolar if the option is available and the patient has a bipolar lead. In some cases surgical intervention may be needed to repair the lead, replace the lead, or change to a bipolar system. See the section on crosstalk below for additional information.

Diaphragm Pacing and Extracardiac Stimulation

This is relatively unusual but may be caused by either an atrial lead stimulating the phrenic nerve or by direct stimulation of the diaphragm or chest wall muscle by the ventricular lead. Extracardiac stimulation occurs due to poor lead placement and/or high output setting of the pacemaker. Occasionally perforation by the lead of the myocardium may cause this as well. Unipolar pacemakers and leads with failed outer insulation may also cause local tissue stimulation.

Corrective Action

Decrease output if possible to do so and still maintain an adequate safety margin for capture. Revision of a culprit lead may be necessary.

Pacemaker Syndrome

This can occur in patients with sinus rhythm who receive VVI pacing systems or in patients with dual chamber devices where the atrial lead does not properly capture or sense. When the atrial contribution to ventricular filling is lost by pacing the ventricle alone, the cardiac output drops and the patient feels fatigued and uncomfortable whenever the pacemaker is pacing. They may have palpitations or chest pulsations due to the "cannon A waves" caused by the atrium contracting against the closed mitral and tricuspid valves. The classic patient to develop pacemaker syndrome is one with retrograde AV node conduction. The latter occurs when the ventricle is paced and contracts. The depolarization impulse travels in a retrograde manner up the bundle of His through the AV node to the atrium. The atrium then contracts against the mitral and tricuspid valves which are closed due to the ventricular contraction. The late atrial contraction causes retrograde blood flow in the venous system with "cannon A waves", dyspnea, fatigue and even syncope. Clues to this phenomenon can be seen on the surface ECG.

In many cases an inverted P-wave can be seen in the T-wave (Fig. 11.7). This represents the retrograde conduction and the ineffective as well as detrimental

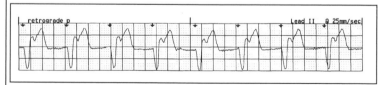

Fig. 11.7. Retrograde conduction. In this example the pacemaker is programmed to VVI. There is a retrogradely conducted and inverted P-wave in the T-wave. This can lead to pacemaker syndrome and pacemaker mediated (endless loop) tachycardia.

atrial contraction. Patients without retrograde conduction may also have a form of pacemaker syndrome due to loss of consistent atrioventricular synchrony. Exacerbating factors predisposing a patient to this problem relate to loss of ventricular compliance. The latter is seen in patients with hypertension, ischemic disease, hypertrophic disease and those who are elderly.

Corrective Action

For VVI devices, reduce the pacing rate or program hysteresis on to allow more time in sinus rhythm. If this does not provide a satisfactory solution, then a change to an atrial or dual chamber device is indicated. If the problem is due to a malfunctioning atrial lead on a dual chamber system, then either reprogram to eliminate the problem or correct the lead surgically.

DUAL CHAMBER PACING

Many pacing problems are shared between single and dual chamber systems. However, there are a number of behaviors and malfunctions that are unique to the dual chamber pacemakers.

PACEMAKER MEDIATED TACHYCARDIA (PMT)

PMT (also referred to as endless loop tachycardia or ELT) is an abnormal state caused by the presence of an accessory pathway (the pacemaker). It is essentially identical to the tachycardia seen in patients with Wolff-Parkinson-White syndrome. PMT often begins with a premature ventricular beat that is either spontaneous or pacemaker induced (Fig 11.8a). The electrical impulse travels retrogradely up the bundle of His to the AV node and then to the atrium (Fig 11.8b). If this retrograde P-wave occurs after PVARP has ended, it will be sensed by the pacemaker. This will start an AV interval, after which the pacemaker will deliver an impulse into the ventricle (Fig 11.8c). This starts the cycle over again. It will continue until one of the following occurs: 1) the retrograde P-wave blocks at the AV node, 2) the retrograde P-wave falls within PVARP, 3) a magnet is applied to the pacemaker (disabling sensing) or 4) the device is reprogrammed to a longer PVARP. The patient may cause transient AV-block by using standard vagal maneuvers to block the AV node terminating the tachycardia. Though not commonly used, adenosine may be given IV to break the tachycardia. PMT may be initiated or restarted by anything that causes a ventricular beat to occur before an atrial beat. This includes a PVC, PJC, loss of atrial sensing or atrial capture, and myopotential tracking or inhibition in the atrium.

PMT may be prevented by appropriate programming of the PVARP such that any retrograde P-waves will fall within this interval and therefore not be sensed by the atrial channel. Unfortunately, in patients with prolonged AV-nodal conduction, the long PVARP that is necessary to prevent PMT may severely limit the

11

maximum tracking rate of the device due to the resulting long TARP. Some pacemakers have special options to prevent PMT, allowing a shorter PVARP to be programmed. One option is the ability to use a short baseline PVARP that automatically extends after any cycle following a sensed R-wave that is not preceded by a P wave (presumably a PVC). This event prolongs the PVARP for only one cycle then reverts back to the shorter one. Another variation of this method is to turn off atrial sensing completely for the cycle following a PVC. This is described as DVI on PVC since there is no atrial sensing for the one cycle. It was once known as DDX by one manufacturer. Finally, some devices provide an automatic termination algorithm if PMT is suspected. When the pacemaker is at its upper rate for a specified number of beats the device may insert a single long PVARP. This action will terminate the PMT if it is present.

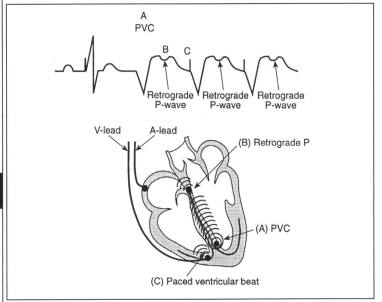

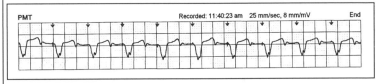

Fig. 11.8. Pacemaker mediated tachycardia (PMT). A PVC occurs (A) causing the ventricle to contract. The electrical impulse is conducted in a retrograde manner through the AV node (B) causing the atrium to contract. The retrograde P wave is sensed by the pacemaker which then starts an AV interval. At the end of the AV interval a pace stimulus is delivered to the ventricle (C) and the cycle continues.

CROSSTALK

This is a potentially dangerous or lethal problem in patients who are pacemaker dependent. Crosstalk occurs when the ventricular sensing amplifier senses the atrial pacing impulse and interprets the atrial pace as an intrinsic ventricular beat. The ventricular output is then inhibited and, if the patient has no ventricular escape, asystole occurs (Fig.11.9). This is seen on the ECG strip as paced atrial P-waves without a ventricular output. Typically the atrial pacing interval is equal to the AEI. This is because the AVI is terminated by the ventricular sensing of the atrial pacing pulse, resetting the pacemaker for the next cycle. However, in an atrial based system the AVI will be allowed to complete before the next AEI starts thus maintaining the programmed pacing rate. Crosstalk is most likely to occur when the atrial output is set very high and the ventricular sensitivity is also set very high.

The prevention of this problem is critical. Most modern pacemakers are very resistant to crosstalk. This problem may be prevented by avoiding settings that predispose the system to crosstalk, and by programming an appropriate blanking period. Additional features may be present to prevent or reduce the effect of crosstalk.

"Safety Pacing" (also known as "Ventricular Safety Standby" and "Non-physiologic AV Delay") allows a brief period of ventricular sensing during the early postatrial output period. This interval that follows the blanking period is known as the "crosstalk sensing window". If an event is sensed in this period of time a ventricular pace is committed at a short AV-delay (usually 100-120 msec). This provides ventricular pacing support should crosstalk actually be present. The ventricular pulse will not fall on the "vulnerable period" should a PVC or other intrinsic atrial beat be present (Fig. 11.10). Please note that this feature does not prevent crosstalk. It is meant only to prevent the result of crosstalk. If safety pacing is present the cause should be identified and corrected as soon as possible.

11

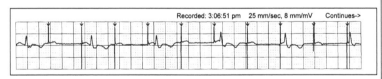

Fig. 11.9. Crosstalk. This pacemkaer is programmed to DDD at 80 bpm with an AVI of 200 ms. Note the paced atrial events with no paced ventricular events and a shorter AA interval. The AEI begins shortly after the atrial pace, advancing the next atrial output by the AVI. This results in a pacing rate above the base rate. If there is no ventricular escape rhythm crosstalk may result in asystole.

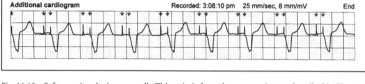

Fig. 11.10a. Safety pacing during crosstalk. This strip is from the same patient as described in Fig. 11.9, however safety pacing is enabled. Instead of paced P waves with no ventricular output, the pacemaker paces at the end of the crosstalk sensing period (see text). The ventricular pace occurs between 110 and 120 msec after the atrial output regardless of the programmed AVI. This feature guards against inappropriate inhibition of the ventricular output.

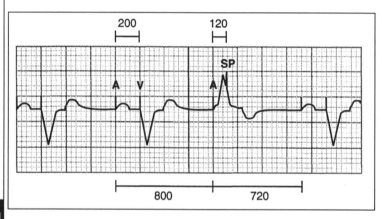

Fig. 11.10b. Safety pacing with PVC. In this example a PVC occurs during the crosstalk sensing period. The pacemaker is not able to differentiate between crosstalk and an actual cardiac event during this period. It therefore will deliver a safety pace (SP). The short AVI used in safety pacing insures that this pulse falls into the refractory period of the ventricle and not onto the vulnerable area of the ST segment.

ACCUFIX/ENCOR LEADS

A unique design for preformed atrial J-leads from Cordis and Telectronics uses a small piece of spring wire either under the insulation of the lead or within the conductor coil(s) of the lead. The purpose of this spring wire is to assist in maintaining the "J" shape of the lead. In a significant number of patients this spring wire has been known to fracture. This can result in perforation of the insulation by the spring wire (Fig. 11.11) with possible perforation of the atrium and even aorta. Should this occur, acute pericardial tamponade could result with a subsequent cardiovascular emergency. Patients with these leads should be screened using cinefluoroscopy in four views to assess the integrity of the lead. If removal of the lead is necesssary or desired, the patient should be referred to a center of excellence.

Figure 11.12 shows a typical lead fracture. Most of these occur as shown in the area just under the clavicle. This is caused by the additional stress placed on the

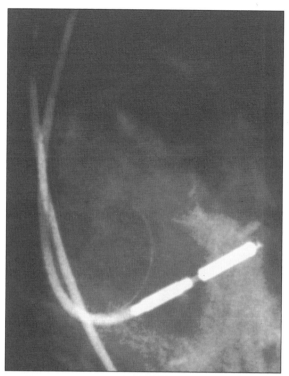

Fig. 11.11. Teletronics Accufix lead radiograph showing fracture and protrusion of the J-retention wire.

11

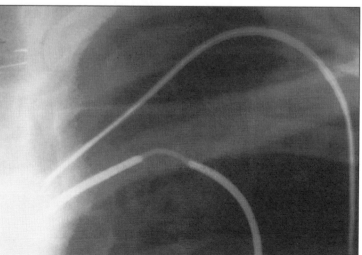

Fig. 11.12. Radiograph of a fractured lead. This lead has a failure of the outer coil as it passes under the clavicle. This is the most common site of lead fracture.

leads as they pass through the soft tissue structures (ligament and muscle) before entering the subclavian vein. Additional stress may be cased by compression of the leads from the first rib and the clavicle when the leads are implanted in a medial postion relative to the first rib. Finally, Figure 11.13 shows a normal appearing PA and lateral chest x-ray. In this example the leads are properly placed into the atrium and ventricle with appropriate amounts of slack in each chamber.

Fig. 11.13. Normal appearing lead placement Radiograph. a. PA radiograph taken with the patient upright with a full inspiration. This is a dual chamber pacemaker with normal appearing lead placement. The atrial lead is in the right atrial appendage and the ventricular lead in the right ventricular apex. The leads have adequate slack, and there are no defects or kinks noted.

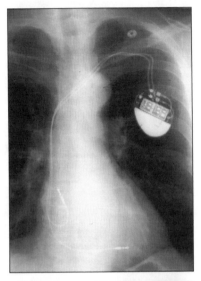

11

Fig. 11.13b. Lateral radiograph of the same patient. Note the anterior position of both leads.

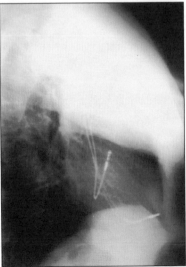

NBD Code for Implantable Cardioverter Defibrillators

The implantable cardioverter defibrillator (ICD) has revolutionized the treatment of lethal tachyarrhythmias. New devices are being designed for the treatment of atrial fibrillation as well. As these devices are quite a bit different in function and have different features than their pacemaker cousins, they need their own descriptive codes. As described in chapter 1, the North American Society of Pacing and Electrophysiology and the British Pacing and Electophysiology Group (NASPE and BPEG or the NBG) developed a system known as the NBG Code to describe the functionality of pacemakers. The fifth position of the code is meant to describe the antitachycardia features of a device. In 1993, the NBG developed another code that was directed at devices whose primary function was that of treating tachycardia rather than bradycardia. This code is very similar to the NBG Code and is known as the NBD Code (NASPE-BPEG Defibrillator Code).

The positions of the NBD code differ in meaning from those of the NBG code, but many of the letters used have the same meanings (Table 12.1). As with the NBG code the first position of the NBD code represents the chamber used for the primary purpose of the device; the delivery of a shock. The chamber(s) shocked are V for Ventricle, A for Atrium, D for Dual and O for no chamber shocked. The second methodology for tachycardia termination is antitachycardia pacing (ATP). The chambers with this type of therapy activated are described by the second position in the code. The letters V, A, D and O used in this position are identical to and have the same meaning as the letters of the first position. The third position describes the method of tachycardia detection. The method for detecting arrhythmias in most antitachycardia devices is the rate and or morphology as seen from the intracardiac electrogram. Another method of detecting an arrhythmia is to monitor a hemodynamic parameter for evidence of compromise or collapse. Therefore E is used to designate Electrogram detection and H is used for Hemodynamic detection. If you remember these first three positions then the last one is easy as it describes the bradycardia pacing capabilities of the defibrillator. This position uses the same letters with the same meaning as the first position of both the NBG and NBD code: V, A, D and O. Some defibrillators have full dual chamber and sensor-driven pacing functions. Complex bradycardia pacing functionality of a defibrillator may be described by adding the first three or four letters of the NBG code after the first three letters of the NBD code. A hyphen is used to separate the two codes for clarity. An example of an ICD that shocks the ventricle with no antitachycardia pacing, uses electrograms for detection and has ventricular bradycardia pacing capability would be described as a VOE-VVI defibrillator.

12

Handbook of Cardiac Pacing, by Charles J. Love. © 1998 Landes Bioscience

Table 12.1. NBD codes (for implantable defibrillators).

1st position indicates the chamber shocked:
V = ventricle
A = atrium
D = dual
O = no shock therapy

2nd position indicates the chamber for antitachycardia pacing:
V = ventricle
A = atrium
D = dual
O = no antitachycardia pacing

3rd position indicates the method of tachycardia detection:
E = electrogram
H = hemodynamic

4th position indicates chambers for bradycardia pacing*
V = ventricle
A = atrium
D = dual
O = no bradycardia pacing.

*Alternatively the three or four letter NBG pacing code may be used following the first three letters of the NBD code (e.g., VVE-VVIR indicating ventricular shock, ventricular ATP, electrogram detection and VVIR pacing capability).

12

The use of two different codes may be a bit confusing. To avoid misunderstanding the code should be followed by the type of device. Examples of this would be "VVEO defibrillator" or "VVIR pacemaker." This implies the NBD and NBG codes respectively. The question as to which code to use if a device has both bradycardia and tachycardia features should be based on the primary design function of the device. An ICD with backup VVI pacing should be described using the NBD format while a pacemaker with antitachycardia pacing capability is best described using the NBG format.

Basic Concepts of Implantable Cardioverter Defibrillators

INTRODUCTION

Though an implantable cardioverter defibrillator (ICD) may look like a large pacemaker and have pacing ability, it is actually quite a different device (Fig. 13.1). The differences are reflected in all aspects of the system from the lead to the power source.

The earliest ICDs were very effective but very primitive relative to today's ICDs and even relative to the pacemakers of the time. The first ICDs were implanted in humans in 1980 and approved for general use by the United States Food and Drug Administration in 1985. These units were similar to the first pacemakers implanted in 1958 as they were not programmable. The device was ordered with a specific detection rate from the factory and no changes were possible other than turning it on or off. This presented significant problems since the patient's arrhythmia substrate is subject to change. Ischemic events, progression of other underlying cardiac disease, and changes in medical therapy may affect tachycardia rates. A common situation would be seen if a new drug such as amiodarone was started on a patient. If the ventricular tachycardia rate were to be slowed below the detection rate of the ICD then the cardioversion would not be delivered as it should have been. The options would be to discontinue the medication or reoperate to replace the ICD using one with a lower detection rate. The cost of an ICD and lead system is in the range of $15,000 to 29,000, and until the recent past required a major surgical procedure. Replacement is not an option that would be done without a great deal of consideration. ICDs that have programmable detection rates have

13

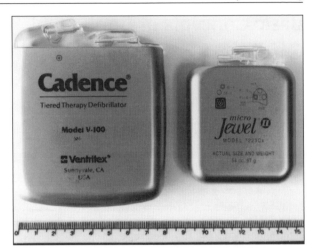

Fig. 13.1a.

Fig. 13.1. Picture of old and new ICDs front (a) and profile (b). Note the marked decrease in size that has occurred over the past 5 years.

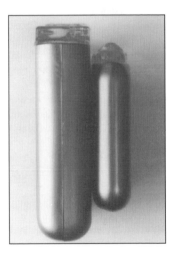

Fig. 13.1b.

been available for general use since 1988. This allows the tailoring of therapy as the patient's needs change.

ICDs subsequently were developed that had several tiers of therapy. Instead of a single detection rate, several detection zones may be set up with different therapy being delivered to the different types of tachycardia. A patient with a history of spontaneous ventricular fibrillation would typically be set to a single zone for detection, and a series of shocks for therapy. Another patient with a history of slow ventricular tachycardia might be set with two zones of therapy. The first zone detects the slow ventricular tachycardia and treats the tachycardia with a series of overdrive pacing pulses. If these are not effective a low energy cardioversion is then performed, and if necessary a high energy shock would be delivered. A second zone to detect faster rates would be entered if the patient still developed spontaneous ventricular fibrillation, rapid ventricular tachycardia, or if in attempting to pace the patient out of the tachycardia the arrhythmia is accelerated. The device would then apply more aggressive therapy and shock the patient immediately. Devices now allow up to four different rate zones for detection. Within each detection zone a series of different therapies are available. There are literally thousands of detection and therapy permutations that may be used. It should be clear that these devices are very complex and that there may be life threatening consequences if programmed improperly. Only persons who are thoroughly familiar with the particular device, the patient's needs, and electrophysiology should prescribe and perform programming changes.

The first ICDs were implanted by opening the chest and placing wire mesh patches directly on the heart or pericardium in order to deliver a high energy shock. Epicardial leads were also placed to sense the heart rate. Multiple approaches to placing the leads on the heart were developed. These included median sternotomy, lateral thoracotomy, subcostal, subxiphod and combinations of these approaches with a transvenous endocardial lead for sensing and pacing the heart. Eventually nonthoracotomy transvenous systems were devised to eliminate the need for opening the chest. These required placing multiple leads in the superior vena cava, subclavian vein, innominate vein and/or the coronary sinus. In many cases a subcutaneous patch or wire array is needed to provide effective therapy. The most advanced devices now combine the ease of using a single lead that combines pacing, sensing and one or more high energy coils for shocking the heart with an "active" or "hot" ICD case that acts as another shocking surface (Fig 13.2). This advanced hardware in combination with more efficient shock waveforms

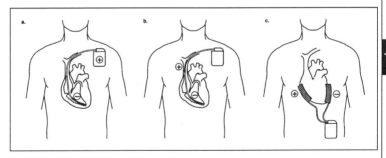

13

Fig. 13.2.a. Active can to coil design is currently the most popular. It is simple in design, easy to implant, and highly effective in converting ventricular arrhythmias. It uses a single coil in the heart (though some systems use an extra coil in the superior vena cava), and the ICD itself is electrically active behaving as the anode or cathode for shock. b. Inactive can and leads is an older design, but still occasionally used, especially for replacement of an existing system of similar design. The ICD itself is not part of the shock circuit. There must therefore be at least 2 coils in the venous system, or 1 coil in the heart and a subcutaneous electrode. c. Epicardial patches and leads are rarely used due to the higher morbidity of the operation, and the high degree of efficacy of the transvenous systems.

has allowed ICD implant to be performed in 30 minutes under local anesthesia as an ambulatory procedure.

BASIC CONCEPTS

Externally the ICD components are the same as those of a pacemaker. Internally there are two major differences.

Battery: The battery of an ICD differs from the chemistry used for pacemakers. The battery of a pacemaker is designed to deliver small amounts of current continuously over many years. The battery in an ICD must deliver large amounts of current in a very short period of time. The chemistry most commonly used is silver vanadium pentoxide. Though the shelf life of this chemistry is not as long as lithium iodine, it has the characteristics needed to provide the current quickly to the capacitors without suffering internal damage. In some cases two batteries may be used in series to improve the charging rate of the capacitors. Newer ICDs are being designed with two types of batteries, one to run the circuitry and pacing functions, and one to charge the capacitors.

CAPACITORS

These large and bulky components are necessary to change the 3 volts supplied by the battery into the 750 volt shock required to defibrillate a heart. Until very recently the basic design of the capacitors had been large and round. This makes them very difficult to place in a space efficient manner in the case. Newer designs using "flat" capacitors and ceramic designs have led to a dramatic decrease in size and much more flexibility in shape. The result is a much smaller case for the components. Capacitors must be charged fully at regular intervals to maintain their ability to charge to full capacity. This is known as "reforming" the capacitor. Earlier devices required that the patient come to the physician's office to charge up the capacitors (without delivering the current to the patient) once every several months. Modern ICDs have an internal clock and calendar that allow the performance of this maintenance function automatically if the patient has not required a shock in several months.

LEAD

The function of the lead system for an ICD includes pacing and sensing the heart as in a standard pacing system. It must also have the ability to deliver approximately 750 volts. In the early designs, different lead systems were used to handle the different functions. One set of leads was present for the sensing and pacing needs and a second set was present for the high energy needs. The latter are shown in Figure 13.3. These would be applied directly to the heart and were placed

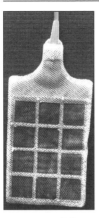

Fig. 13.3a. Originally, large patches such as this once were placed directly on the surface of the heart. Later, they were also used subcutaneously to provide additional surface area for transvenously placed systems.

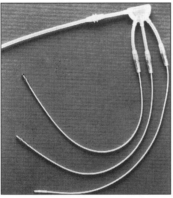

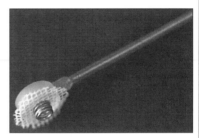

Fig. 13.3c (above). Screw on electrodes were used to pace and sense the heart. These are designed to be placed on the epicardial surface of the heart and were used in most of the implants before the transvenous systems were introduced.

Fig. 13.3b (above). As a variant on the patch, a subcutaneous array was developed. These coils were inserted into the tissues between the ribs.

13

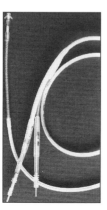

Fig. 13.3d. Transvenous electrodes have virtually replaced all epicardial lead systems for ICDs. They are placed in a manner similar to pacing leads.

within the central venous circulation, in the great cardiac vein, or in the subcutaneous tissue. The sensing leads were epicardial screw-in or in some cases were long pacing leads placed transvenously. As with pacing leads, conductor fractures and insulation failures are not uncommon.

SENSING

Sensing the heart rate is very important as this is the primary method for the ICD to determine if a tachycardia is present or not. There are two configurations that are true bipolar and integrated bipolar. True bipolar sensing uses the same methodology as in pacing. A lead with the cathode and anode are present within the ventricle (Fig 13.4a). These are dedicated to pacing and sensing functions and do not form any part of the shocking high voltage circuit. The second configuration uses a cathode at the tip; however the anode is the distal shocking coil (Fig 13.4b). This configuration is referred to as "integrated bipolar," allowing the lead to be of more simple design. However, since the shock coil doubles as the sensing coil there may be some difficulty sensing immediately after a shock is delivered. This rapidly resolves and normal sensing resumes. Some devices use true bipolar sensing and integrated bipolar pacing to overcome this limitation.

Due to the possible extreme differences in intracardiac electrograms between normal beats, premature ventricular beats and ventricular fibrillation, the standard sensing methods used in pacing do not work well in ICDs. The fixed sensitivity level is not able to adapt to these wide swings in electrogram size. Most ICDs use some variation of automatic gain control. After each sensed event the sensitivity is decreased, after which the device becomes increasingly more sensitive. This helps to prevent oversensing of noncardiac events and the evoked T-wave. The longer the device goes without sensing an event, the more sensitive it becomes. This function provides the ability to detect if the patient has gone into a fine ventricular fibrillation that might otherwise be missed if the sensitivity was not so high.

13

Fig 13.4a. True bipolar sensing occurs between a cathode and anode separate from the defibirillation coils. b. Integrated bipolar sensing uses a cathode on the lead with one of the defibrilation coils as the sensing anode. Sensing may not be quite as reliable compared with the true bipolar configuration.

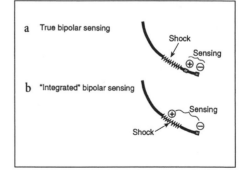

DETECTION

The most straightforward method of determining if an arrhythmia is present is to use a simple rate criteria. This is very sensitive, but lacks specificity. In other words, it will sense virtually all life threatening arrhythmias but may also detect sinus tachycardia or atrial fibrillation with a rapid ventricular response. In order to improve the specificity of arrhythmia, additional detection parameters may be used. These are listed in Table 13.1. It must be remembered that as with any test, increasing the specificity means decreasing the sensitivity. I always say that it is better to have an angry patient calling me due to an unnecessary shock rather than not to have a patient alive due to failure of the algorithm to detect a lethal arrhythmia. For this reason, the additional detection criteria are available to modify the lower ventricular tachycardia zones and NOT the ventricular fibrillation zone.

The rate stability criteria is useful when a patient has atrial fibrillation with a rapid ventricular response at times. If the ventricular tachycardia detection rate and the ventricular rate when the patient is in atrial fibrillation overlap, then the patient could get an unnecessary shock or series of shocks. Ventricular tachycardia tends to be very regular beat to beat while the ventricular response to atrial fibrillation tends to be very irregular. The rate stability criteria allows the programming of a beat to beat variability limit (Fig 13.5). If the rhythm varies more than this amount, it is classified as not being ventricular tachycardia and therapy is withheld. The shortcomings of this methodology would be the presence of a

---

Table 13.1. Detection criteria

Rate only
Rate stability
Sudden rate onset
Sustained high rate
Morphology
Atrial rhythm discrimination

13

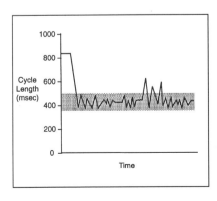

Fig. 13.5. Rate stability may be used in addition to the ventricular rate as a secondary factor to determine the type of arrhythmia that is present. While ventricular tachycardia tends to be quite regular, fast ventricular rates caused by atrial fibrillation with a rapid ventricular response tend to be irregular. This diagram shows a situation where the ventricular tachycardia detection zone is set between 500 ms and 350 ms, and the ventricular fibrillation zone is below 350 ms. Though the heart rate is in the VT zone, it is quite irregular, and thus may be due to atrial fibrillation. The device can be programmed to not deliver pace or shock therapy in this situation.

polymorphic ventricular tachycardia which would not be regular like monomorphic ventricular tachycardia. The polymorphic types tend to be faster in rate and thus are less likely to overlap with the rates as seen in atrial fibrillation.

Another type of problem patient is one who is physically active and has a slow ventricular tachycardia. In this case the sinus rates may overlap with the slow ventricular tachycardia detection zone. In order to avoid shocking the patient when the rate enters the detection zone due to normal activity, a sudden onset criteria may be used. Sinus tachycardia tends to enter the detection zone in a gradual manner with the heart rate slowly accelerating into the detection zone. Ventricular tachycardia tends to enter the detection zone rapidly, often after a premature ventricular beat. The sudden onset criteria requires that if the interval between the beat just before entry into the detection zone and the beat that is in the detection zone be longer than a specified period of time (Fig 13.6).

Since it is possible for ventricular tachycardia to occur and be missed due to the use of the algorithms, another criteria may be activated to act as a backup system. This is known as "sustained high rate," "extended high rate" and "sustained rate duration." They are all basically the same, though each manufacturer calls it by a different name. The purpose of this feature is to activate the therapy if the rate stays in the detection zone for a prolonged period of time. Since it is possible for a patient to enter the tachycardia zone slowly by exercising and then develop ventricular tachycardia or for a patient to have a ventricular tachycardia with an irregular rate, this feature acts as a "safety net". It works by delivering therapy if it had been withheld after a specified period of time or number of beats.

Fig. 13.6. Sudden onset of a fast rate may be used to differentiate VT from sinus tachycardia. VT tends to start with a PVC and thus an abrupt change in cycle length is noted (13.6a). Sinus tachycardia tends to shorten the cycle length gradually (13.6b). The tachycardia shown in (a) will be treated while the one in (b) will not be treated.

13

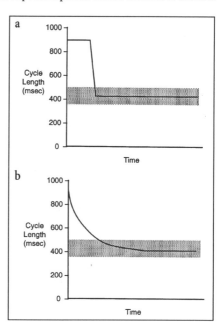

When a clinician attempts to determine whether a rhythm is ventricular tachycardia or supraventricular tachycardia the width of the QRS if often quite helpful. Wide complex beats are most often ventricular and narrow complex beats are usually supraventricular in origin. The ICD may use a morphology criteria to determine whether a beat is wide or narrow. This differentiation may not work in patients with underlying bundle branch block, rate dependent bundle branch block or narrow morphology ventricular tachycardia. It does work in other patients and may be used alone or with one of the other criteria in addition to the detection rate.

The newest discrimination method to be introduced is the use of the intracardiac atrial signal as compared with the ventricular signal. The presence of atrioventricular dissociation is diagnostic of a primary ventricular rhythm. Using this technique a relatively slow ventricular rate that is present with an even slower atrial rate can be assumed to be ventricular tachycardia as opposed to sinus tachycardia. In addition, the atrial lead may be able to detect a rapid atrial rate to determine that the fast irregular ventricular rate is more likely to be due to atrial fibrillation with a rapid ventricular response. Obviously one must be very cautious when making these determinations.

DEFIBRILLATION WAVEFORM

Just as with pacemaker pulses, the defibrillation pulse has both an amplitude and a duration. The initial type of shock waveform was the monophasic truncated exponential shape (Fig 13.7a). This delivered the energy in one direction. Though this was effective in many patients it was not always successful. It was even less effective when being used with the nonthoracotomy configurations. The newer devices virtually all use a biphasic waveform (Fig 13.7b). During the delivery of energy with a biphasic pulse the initial direction of the current is reversed.

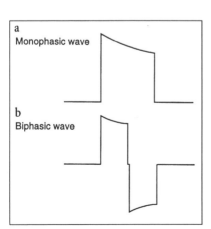

a
Monophasic wave

b
Biphasic wave

Fig. 13.7a. This is a diagram of a truncated exponential monophasic waveform. This was the standard waveform of the early ICDs, and is still used in virtually all external defibrillators. b. The biphasic waveform as shown has been found to be significanly more effective than the monophasic version for converting fibrillating heart rhythms to normal in most patients. It has allowed the devices to be smaller due to the lower DFTs achieved.

13

This has been found to be an excellent method of defibrillation, and for the majority of patients results in a significantly lower amount of energy required to restore the normal heart rhythm. Not only is polarity of the pulse important, but the duration of the pulse (if monophasic) or duration of each segment of the pulse (if biphasic) is critical. Pulses that are too short or too long will not be effective. Pulses that spend too much time in one phase versus the other phase will likewise be less effective.

DEFIBRILLATION THRESHOLD

Unlike pacing where the threshold is a fairly reproducible point on a strength duration curve, the defibrillation threshold in a given patient with a given system is a probability. A probability curve as shown in Figure 13.8 can theoretically be produced for each patient. Unfortunately, given the method of device implant this is rarely done. Typically two successful defibrillations at a single energy level are used to confirm that the device will work. Some implantors will do repeated testing until the lowest energy level that still defibrillates is found. Though this seems much like pacemaker threshold testing, it is not. Without extensive and repeated testing, the shape and position of the defibrillation threshold probability curve will not be known. For practical purposes, the two shock method gives a relatively high probability of being above the 90% confidence level for conversion of ventricular fibrillation at a given energy level.

ANTI-TACHYCARDIA PACING (ATP)

ATP Is a very useful method to terminate monomorphic ventricular tachycardia. It is most commonly used for slow tachycardias and those for which the patient is hemodynamically stable. The principle behind ATP is to entrain the tachycardia by pacing at a rate faster than the tachycardia. This can allow the electrical circuit within the myocardium that is perpetuating the rhythm to fatigue or block. In either case the tachycardia terminates (Fig. 13.9). Patients find this method of

Fig. 13.8. DFT Probability curve. Defibrillation is not an absolute occurrence. At high energy levels there is still the possibility that the delivered energy may not restore normal rhythm. Conversely, at low energy levels there ay still be a small chance that defibrillation will occur. To insure that a single defibrillation was not a lucky conversion in the low probability zone, several tests of the system need to be performed in order to verify that the subsequent probability of rescue is high.

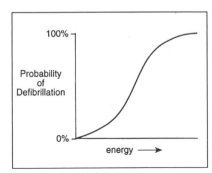

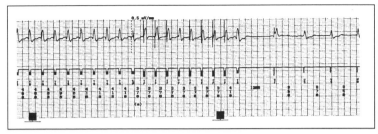

Fig. 13.9. ATP success. This patient went into ventricular tachycardia at a cycle length of 400-410 ms. The ICD delivers 8 paced pulses at 370 ms which terminates the arrhythmia. The top trace is a far field electrogram recording from the shock electrode and defibrillator case, bottom trace shows the events as noted and telemetered by the defibrillator (TS=tachycardia sense, TD=tachycardia detected, TP=anti-tachycardia pacing, VP=ventricular pace, VS=ventricular sense). The numbers are the intervals measured between events.

arrhythmia termination far more preferable than receiving a shock. The most common way of delivering the ATP is by the device measuring the cycle length of the tachycardia. It then will deliver a short burst of pacing pulses that begin at some percentage (e.g., 87%) of the tachycardia cycle length. The pace pulses may all be at one cycle length, or there may be a progressive shortening between each pulse. The latter is known as RAMP pacing and is more effective than the fixed interval burst type. One concern that is present when using ATP is the possibility of accelerating the tachycardia or fibrillating the heart. Should either one of these happen the next level of therapy is available to deliver a cardioversion or defibrillation. ATP is rarely programmed on as a sole therapy without shock therapy as a backup. Another issue that must be considered is that ATP may cause a substantial delay in the delivery of definitive therapy. This is usually not a problem except in patients with ischemic cardiac disease. These patients may become severely ischemic during long courses of ineffective ATP and be less likely to be successfully defibrillated if not done so quickly. Thus, ATP is indicated in patients with hemodynamically stable ventricular tachycardia that has demonstrated termination with overdrive pacing. It should be avoided in those patients where acceleration of the tachycardia or induction of fibrillation has been shown to occur. It should not be used in patients with hemodynamically unstable rhythms.

13

COMMITTED VS. NONCOMMITTED

Once the ICD has detected a rhythm for which it is to deliver a shock there are two possible courses of action. The first is to simply charge to the programmed output and deliver the shock. This is referred to as a committed shock as once detection occurs the device is committed to deliver therapy. The second possibility is for the device to recheck or take a second look at the rhythm either while it is charging or just before it delivers the shock. This is referred to as noncommitted since the ICD can "change it's mind." The advantage to a noncommitted device is that if the tachycardia turns out to be a nonsustained event the ICD will not deliver an unnecessary shock. However, we are again faced with improving the specificity at the expense of sensitivity. In withholding the shock it is possible that due to low amplitude fibrillation waves or polymorphic tachycardia that the ICD might miss detecting the tachycardia on the second look. Most devices allow for the first shock to be programmed as committed or noncommitted with the remainder of the shocks being committed. The choice of which way to set the device is left to the physician. Patients with a history of nonsustained ventricular tachycardia or atrial fibrillation with periods of rapid response will typically have the noncommitted shock feature on. Those with paroxysmal ventricular fibrillation will often have it set to committed to insure that a shock is not delayed.

BRADYCARDIA BACKUP AND POSTSHOCK PACING

Virtually all ICDs being implanted have the ability to pace the ventricle as a VVI pacemaker would. They may have a single pacing rate, a hysteresis rate and/or a postshock pacing rate. The ability to pace VVI may be present even if ATP is not available. Though pacing is available it is not routinely used as the primary source of rate support for patients who require a pacemaker as well as an ICD. This is due to the significant impact that sustained pacing can have on device longevity. It may reduce the expected life of the ICD by up to 50% making it a very expensive pacemaker. If pacing is going to be needed on a regular basis then a separate dedicated pacemaker is frequently used. Some ICDs have two levels of pacing output. One is used for routine bradycardia pacing and the other for ATP and postshock pacing. The postshock and ATP outputs are typically set higher due to the possibility of higher thresholds when the patient may be hypoxemic, acidemic and ischemic. The postshock settings are typically used for several minutes before the standard settings are restored. Some ICDs also allow the programming of a postshock pause before pacing starts and for a separate postshock pacing rate. ICDs with full DDD capability are now available. DDDR capability will be introduced in the near future as well.

COUNTERS AND ELECTROGRAMS

The most vital function that the device can serve other that rescuing the patient from a cardiac arrest is to assist the clinician in determining the etiology of the event to which the device responded. Early ICDs had a simple counter that indicated the number of device charges and discharges. This was only useful to determine if a shock had occurred. There were no data recorded regarding the rate of the arrhythmia, the date or time of occurrence, or the morphology of the

QRS at the time. The first improvement was the addition of a data logging system that detailed the date and time of the arrhythmia and even of nonsustained events. This was combined with a memory that would show the cycle lengths of the rhythm (Fig 13.10). By reviewing this information, decisions regarding the type of arrhythmia could be inferred. Regular intervals were consistent with monomorphic ventricular tachycardia, while irregular intervals were assumed to be polymorphic ventricular tachycardia, atrial fibrillation with a rapid ventricular response, or with ventricular fibrillation if the intervals were short enough. If the intervals were excessively short, one would consider electromagnetic interference or a lead failure that generated false signals (fractures and insulation failures can cause this). ICDs are now capable of recording the intracardiac electrogram or a "far field" electrogram during tachycardia detection and therapy. The "far field" electrogram is recorded from electrodes that are not those typically used for sensing. This is done by using the two shocking surfaces or a combination of shocking surface and intracardiac electrode (the typical sensing electrode). The difference between the near field and far field signals is shown in Figure 13.11. Note that the appearance of the QRS and even the P-wave of the far field electrogram and the similarity of this complex to that of a surface ECG recording. This is very useful to see what the atrial activity is during the arrhythmia. Most devices do not begin to record electrograms until tachycardia is detected. Some devices have a function available similar to the looping memory event recorders. These ICDs are constantly recording the electrograms and are able to freeze this information in memory when a tachycardia starts. This not only gives a picture of the arrhythmia, but also creates a record of the initiation of the event. Information of this type is very valuable to the clinician but very expensive in terms of battery drain. This feature is usually turned off unless there is a need to use it for diagnostic purposes.

```
Date Interrogated: Nov 05, 1997  13:55:20
Date Last Cleared: Apr 30, 1997  12:57:24

DATE           TIME       TYPE    STATUS
Oct 07, 1997   14:44:10   VT      VT Rx 1 Successful
Oct 05, 1997   15:25:43   VT      VT Rx 1 Successful
Oct 05, 1997   14:21:57   VT      VT Rx 1 Successful
Oct 04, 1997   23:57:12   VT      VT Rx 1 Successful
Oct 02, 1997   18:52:27   VT      VT Rx 1 Successful
```

Fig. 13.10. The data log is a key element of the ICD evaluation. It details the date and time of each event that met the detection criteria of the ICD, and the action taken by the device.

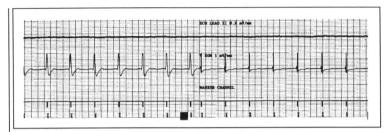

Fig. 13.11. Near and far field signals. The first group of complexes are recorded between the distal shock coil and the defibrillator case. These are referred to as "far field" because they are distant to the intraventricular sensing electrodes. The second group of complexes are recorded from the sensing electrodes within the right ventricle. These are referred to as "near field".

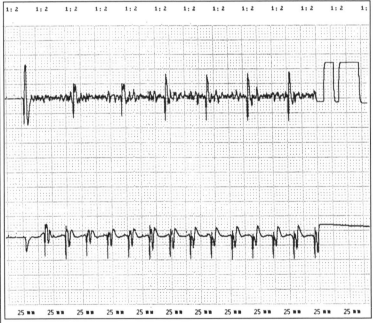

Fig. 13.12. Atrial and ventricular intracardiac signals. This is a tracing from a patient in ventricular tachycardia. The top tracing is an intracardiac atrial electrogram with a sinus rate of around 105 bpm. The bottom trace is an intracardiac ventricular electrogram showing a rate of 200 bpm. This is classic AV dissociation, with the ventricle going faster than the atrium and is diagnostic of ventricular tachycardia. It rules out atrial fibrillation, atrial flutter or supraventricular tachycardia as the cause for the rapid ventricular rate.

MAGNET RESPONSE OF THE ICD

ICDs have a very different response to magnet application than do pacemakers. In addition, the effect of sustained magnet application may differ from one device to another and may even be programmable as to the effect of the magnet. There is one feature that is constant across all ICDs with magnet application which is the suspension of tachycardia therapy. If a patient is receiving inappropriate shocks or if for any reason suspending therapy becomes necessary, placing a ring type pacemaker magnet over the ICD will immediately prevent further therapy from being delivered. Some devices can be programmed to the "off" setting by keeping the magnet in place for 30 seconds. The latter type of device can be turned back "on" by placing the magnet over it for 30 seconds as well. Others will immediately resume detection and therapy when the magnet is removed no matter how long the magnet has been applied. This is a useful feature when a programmer is not available. Though the tachycardia therapy is disabled by the magnet, the bradycardia backup pacing remains active. Thus, if the patient has no heart rhythm without the backup pacing of the defibrillator, there will still be rhythm support during magnet application. To make things a bit more confusing, some ICDs have a programmable magnet feature. This allows the magnet effect to be ignored by the device.

RECOMMENDED REPLACEMENT TIME

Unlike pacemakers where the magnet rate signals the need for device replacement there is no simple method to determine battery life on an ICD. At least two manufacturers allow the programming of a beeping tone that sounds regularly when the battery gets low. For most devices the routine follow-up in the clinic provides telemetry that indicates the battery voltage and the time it takes to charge the capacitors to their full voltage. When either one of these gets to a specified value, then it is time to replace the device. Most ICDs can now be expected to last between 4 to 7 years in normal use.

13

Indications for Implantable Cardioverter Defibrillators

Implantable defibrillators represent a quantum leap in our ability to prevent recurrent sudden cardiac death due to ventricular dysrhythmias. These devices recognize rapid heart rates and are capable of delivering overdrive pacing, cardioversion, or defibrillation therapy. The original implants were performed using a thoracotomy. Newer systems are placed in a transvenous manner allowing patients to leave the hospital after 24 hours. The effectiveness of these devices exceeds 95% over several years. In general, an ICD should be used when a patient is at high risk for recurrent life threatening arrhythmias when no other effective therapy is available, reliable, or tolerated to prevent a sudden death event. Situations that are preventable such as digitalis toxicity with hypokalemia do not justify ICD insertion. The current guidelines as published by the American College of Cardiology and the American Heart Association are as follows:

CLASS I: GENERAL AGREEMENT THAT AN ICD IS INDICATED

Primary VT or VF not due to a transient or reversible cause (drug toxicity, acute myocardial infarction, electrolyte disturbance, etc.)

Spontaneous sustained VT

Syncope of uncertain cause with inducible poorly tolerated sustained ventricular tachycardia or ventricular fibrillation (clinically relevant) at EP study in a patient whom no effective, tolerated, or preferred drug is found during testing.

Spontaneous nonsustained VT in a patient post myocardial infarction when inducible VT or VF is found that is not suppressed by a class-1 antiarrhythmic drug

14

CLASS II: SOME DISAGREEMENT AS TO THE NECESSITY FOR IMPLANT

A: WEIGHT OF EVIDENCE IN FAVOR OF EFFICACY
None

B: EFFICACY LESS WELL ESTABLISHED BY WEIGHT OF EVIDENCE

Cardiac arrest due to VF when electrophysiologic testing is not possible due to medical reasons

Symptomatic VT or VF in a patient awaiting cardiac transplantation

Familial or inherited conditions that place the patient at high risk (e.g. long QT syndrome or hypertrophic myopathy)

Spontaneous nonsustained VT in a patient post myocardial infarction when inducible VT or VF is found during electrophysiology study

Recurrent syncope of uncertain cause in the presence of LV dysfunction, inducible VT or VF at electophysiology study, and no other cause of syncope is found

CLASS III

Recurrent syncope of uncertain cause in a patient without inducible ventricular tachycardia or ventricular fibrillation

Incessant ventricular tachycardia or ventricular fibrillation

Ventricular tachycardia or ventricular fibrillation due to a reversible cause such as drug, metabolic or ischemic conditions

VT due to an arrhythmia amenable to catheter ablation or surgical therapy

Significant psychiatric illness that may prevent proper follow-up of the device, or which may be adversely affected by a device implant

Terminal illness or life expectancy less than 6 months

Patients with LV dysfunction, prolonged QRS, absence of spontaneous or inducible VT or VF, who are undergoing coronary bypass surgery

NYHA class IV in patients that are not candidates for heart transplantation

14

ADDITIONAL ISSUES FOR ICD INSERTION

Patient life expectancy should be greater than 6 months

The patient should be emotionally stable

The patient should be willing and able to cooperate in follow-up

Heart failure greater than NYHA Class III should contraindicate an ICD implant unless it is being used as a "bridge" to heart transplantation.

Recently the results of a multicenter trial known as MADIT were published. This was the Multicenter Automatic Defibrillator Implant Trial. The trial was based on the knowledge that patients with recent myocardial infarction, residual ejection fraction of 35% or less, and spontaneous non-sustained ventricular tachycardia were at high risk for sudden arrhythmic death. The patients were evaluated by electrophysiolgy study. Those that had inducible but non suppressed ventricular tachycardia had a significantly better survival if they were treated prophylactically with an ICD as opposed to medical therapy. This prophylactic reason for implantation of an ICD has recently been adapted as an indication. The evidence is quite strong that this well defined group of patients will benefit from having an ICD implanted.

14

Preoperative, Operative and Postoperative Considerations for Implantable Cardioverter Defibrillators

INTRODUCTION

Implantion of ICDs has become much easier with the advent of the smaller, active can, biphasic waveform devices combined with efficient defibrillation lead systems. As previously noted, ICD implants originally required an open chest procedure or at the least a subxiphoid approach to enter the pericardium and place patches and screw-in leads directly onto the myocardium. The preoperative and postoperative issues for this type of procedure were far more involved as was the recovery time for the patient. Mortality and morbidity rates were significant from the longer and more invasive approach. As greater than 99% of ICDs are implanted in a subcutaneous manner with transvenous leads, the following discussion will be focused on this less invasive approach.

PREOPERATIVE PATIENT ISSUES

We approach the preoperative management of the patient who is about to receive an ICD in much the same way as we do the patient who is going to receive a pacemaker (see chapter 10). The patient is first given information about the ICD and the reason the device was recommended. It is very important to stress that the ICD will NOT prevent the tachycardia. This is a common patient misconception. It must be clear that the device is meant only to correct the arrhythmia once it occurs. Though many patients may be able to reduce or discontinue their antiarrhythmia medication, some patients may still require drug therapy to reduce the frequency of tachycardia. The patient should be allowed to see and hold a model of the ICD. This helps provide a perspective of what the incision and

15

physical appearance of the implant area will look like. A description of the lead system and the operation is provided. The fact that the patient will have the ICD tested several times during the procedure should be discussed. The possibility that death may occur should be raised with an emphasis on the benefits of the procedure relative to the risks. Due to the size of the ICD and the lack of true surgical training of some physicians who implant them, infections are more frequent than with pacemakers. The larger size of the device may compromise blood flow to the adjacent tissues creating local ischemia. This may result in an erosion or predisposition to infection.

The preparation of the patient is identical to that for a permanent pacemaker. However, some physicians prefer the use of general anesthesia for ICD implant. This may be a preference for all patients or only for selected cases where the patient may require more aggressive sedation. In some cases the patient may be at very high risk due to compromised cardiovascular or pulmonary disease. Cases such as these should be done with prior consultation of an anesthesiologist. It is important to be sure that this consultant understands the nature of the procedure. We have had cases where lidocaine was administered by the anesthetist when recurrent ventricular ectopy was observed during our attempts to induce ventricular fibrillation. It is somewhat difficult for an anesthesiologist who spends his time trying to keep the patient out of harm's way to accept the intentional acts of the electrophysiologist who wants to fibrillate the ventricle.

SURGICAL CONSIDERATIONS

The implant has been greatly simplified with the advent of active can, biphasic, small defibrillators. Patch placement directly on the myocardium or on the pericardium via median sternotomy, left lateral thoracotomy, subxiphoid or subcostal approaches has been virtually eliminated. Single transvenous lead implants are successful 95-98% of the time without the use of subcutaneous patches, subcutaneous arrays or additional transvenous leads.

In the operating room the following sequence of events takes place. First all of the equipment is checked for proper operation. The patient is sedated and the lead is implanted. The lead is tested for routine pacing capture and sensing thresholds. A pocket is made for the ICD which is attached to the lead. A low energy shock is delivered through the high voltage ends to verify the electrical connections. The patient is then further sedated if necessary and ventricular fibrillation is induced. A simple method commonly used is to choose a moderate shock energy level around 15 to 20 joules. If the patient can be converted twice with this amount of energy then the incision is closed. Other physicians prefer to determine the actual defibrillation threshold (DFT). This may be done by repeatedly fibrillating the patient and reducing the shock energy to a level that no longer defibrillates the patient. The patient is then rescued internally or externally. Unless we are doing an investigational lead or ICD that requires testing of this type, we prefer the rapid method. The patient may be returned to a telemetry unit and may be discharged the following day if the postoperative evaluation and chest x-ray are acceptable.

Additional postoperative patient care will be dictated by the surgical approach. In some cases, where a thoracotomy is performed a chest tube will be present. The cardiovascular status should be monitored closely, especially in patients who have undergone extensive DFT testing. Pulmonary care, early mobilization and emotional support may also be necessary.

PREDISCHARGE QUESTIONS AND ISSUES

Virtually all of the postoperative issues addressed in the pacing section apply to patients with an ICD implant. However there is one subject that will consistently cause the most anxiety for both the patient and the physician: driving. There are several issues that must be addressed regarding the operation of motor vehicles. The first consideration is what the law requires. This is very confusing and will vary significantly from state to state. Some states have no requirements while others may have mandatory license suspensions for up to two years following an arrhythmic event resulting in a loss of consciousness. In some states the physician is obligated to notify the Bureau of Motor Vehicles, and in others the physician is forbidden from doing so to prevent an invasion of the patient's right to privacy.

The approach that I use is practical when the law is unclear or does not cover these situations. If the patient has had an arrhythmic event where loss of control or syncope has occurred they are to abstain from driving for 6 months. If no further events occur in this period of time they may drive again unless they are deemed to be at excessive risk. Otherwise I permit them to resume driving in 4 weeks. These cautions also apply to the use of machinery, lawn mowing equipment and working on heights. Some patients will ask if they can "just drive around town but stay off of the highway." My answer to that is that my children play in the front yard. The patient is more likely to injure someone else or have a property damage accident in the city. The abstinence from driving is consistently the most difficult part of the patient's situation with which the physician or nurse must deal. In our clinic we make a point of telling the patient that it is not the ICD that is preventing them from driving. It is the fact that they have a cardiac arrhythmia. This removes inappropriate anger directed at the ICD and allows the patient to accept the device more easily. It is often useful to compare the arrhythmia patient to the patient with epilepsy. Seizure patients also have to deal with periodic loss of consciousness and driving restrictions related to their disease.

15

EMERGENCY CARE OF PATIENTS WITH AN ICD

Standard emergency procedures should always be initiated for ICD patients in ventricular tachycardia or fibrillation. This includes the initiation of standard Basic Cardiac Life Support and Advance Cardiac Life Support procedures as indicated. If initial anterior and lateral external electrical countershock is not successful, repositioning the paddles to the anterior and posterior position may be helpful. If in physical contact with patient when the ICD discharges one may feel a slight tingle. Though this may be felt by the rescuer it will not be harmful. If rubber or latex gloves are worn then no electrical current will be felt by the rescuer.

Evaluation of Defibrillator Malfunction

EVALUTION OF DEFIBRILLATOR MALFUNCTION

When an ICD malfunctions or repeated shocks are delivered to the patient, a life threatening or very uncomfortable situation may occur. Failure of an ICD to deliver a shock when it should can result in death or prolonged episodes of ventricular tachycardia. Delivering inappropriate shocks to the patient is very painful and can possibly induce an arrhythmia. As clinicians we most often see patients due to inappropriate shocks. This is an obvious problem for the patient, and they will call the clinic or come to the emergency department. If a device fails to shock we would at best see the patient due to a sustained arrhythmia. The worst scenario would be failure to shock ventricular fibrillation with subsequent death of the patient. In the latter situation we might not even know of the death until the patient fails to show for the next clinic visit.

Since virtually all of the ICDs available in the market now have anti-bradycardia pacing capability they are subject to virtually all of the same problems as pacemakers. Please refer to the chapter on evaluation of pacemaker malfunction for a review of these issues. The same leads that provide pacing and sensing functions for the bradycardia section of the ICD also provide the sensing function for the tachycardia detection. In the case of "integrated bipolar" systems, one of the shocking electrodes functions as the sensing and pacing anode as well. Although it is possible to evaluate the impedance of the pacing portion of the system in a noninvasive and painless manner, we are not yet able to do the same for the high voltage portion of the circuit. Most ICDs will measure the high voltage impedance when a shock is delivered. To do this requires that the patient have had a spontaneous device discharge. If this has not occurred, a manual discharge may be delivered. Most patients are not too willing to have this done on a routine basis. This makes evaluation of the entire system difficult during a routine clinic follow-up.

16

The approach to the patient with a suspected ICD malfunction is essentially the same as the approach to the pacemaker patient. Gathering the basic data concerning the ICD, patient disease, indications for the device implant, and circumstances surrounding the incident in question are all essential. Interrogation of the ICD with all of the available telemetry is also required. Many times the issue is whether or not a device discharge was appropriate or not. On devices with limited diagnostic capability the history surrounding the shock is crucial. If the patient felt palpitations, lightheaded, short of breath or had syncope, then the discharge was likely delivered for the right reasons. However, the absence of these symptoms does not mean that the shock was not proper. In many cases the patient may be sitting or may be supine and is not sufficiently hypotensive for a long enough period of time to become symptomatic. In other cases the patient may simply not remember the event since they were not perfusing their brain at the time. If the ICD detected and treated the arrhythmia quickly there may have been insufficient time for symptoms to occur. Occasionally the patient may even have been sleeping at the time of the arrhythmia. Indeed, nocturnal myoclonus is frequently misinterpreted by the patient's spouse as a device discharge.

The most common problem in our clinic is not really an ICD problem but a response to the arrhythmia atrial fibrillation. If atrial fibrillation occurs with a rapid ventricular response that exceeds the detection rate of the device, the ICD will charge and shock the patient. It may even do so numerous times. Occasionally the shock will convert the atrial fibrillation to sinus rhythm; however, this does not happen on a regular basis. These shocks do not represent a device malfunction, though the situation is best described as an undesirable patient-device interaction.

The specific categories of device malfunction are noted below. Suggestions as to how to manage these problems follow each section.

FAILURE TO SHOCK OR DELIVER ANTI-TACHYCARDIA PACING

The failure of an ICD to deliver anti-tachycardia therapy can be lethal. The reasons for failure to shock are listed in Table 16.1. The two most common reasons for failure to deliver therapy that we see are lead failure and a detection rate that is too high. Unfortunately, lead failures are not uncommon. Some types of failure are visible on a X-ray but many are not. The fracture may occur on one of the inner conductors of a coaxial or triaxial lead. If this happens the outer conductor may shield the inner conductor from being seen on X-ray. Other fractures may occur that result in the two broken ends remaining in contact at times and being apart at other times. These are also difficult to see by radiography. Figure 16.1 shows failure of epicardial patches with the conductor broken where it meets the

Fig. 16.1. (opposite page) Radiograph of a patch failure. Epicardial screw in leads are noted as well as the patches. Note the discontinuity between the lead and the patch (arrows). This system was nonfunctional and required replacement with a transvenous system.

Table 16.1. Failure to shock

Undersensing
Lead malposition
Lead dislodgment
Lead perforation
Lead fracture
Lead insulation failure
Lead to device connector problem
Sensitivity set too low (i.e., insensitive)
Poor electrogram amplitude due to change in myocardial substrate
Myocardial infarction
Drug therapy
Metabolic imbalance
"Fine" ventricular fibrillation
Primary circuit failure
Battery failure
Shock therapy turned off (by programming or magnet)
Magnet placed over the device
Strong magnetic field present
Detection rate set too high
Failure to meet additional detection criteria
    Rate stability
    Sudden onset
    Morphology criteria
Slowing of tachycardia below detection rate
Electrolyte changes
Drug therapy changes
Interaction with permanent pacemaker

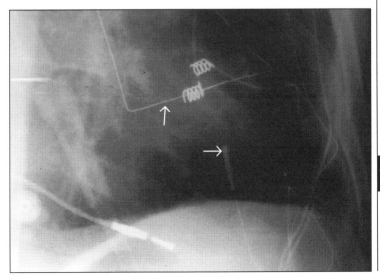

16

patch. This is a common site of patch failure and should be looked for when evaluating the X-ray. Several views may be required to visualize the failure. An overpenetrated film is better for seeing wire failures. We find it best to ask the radiology department to use a "thoracic spine technique" when determining the exposure settings on our chest films.

If the undersensing problem develops within 30 days after implant then lead malposition, dislodgment or myocardial perforation should be suspected. Fractures and insulation failures are more likely to occur after one or more years. As the transvenous defibrillation leads, are substantially thicker than pacing leads they are exposed to more forces under the clavicle when placed by the popular subclavian access technique. This is the area to pay special attention to when reviewing the x-ray. Observation of the connector pins within the connector block of the ICD will reveal an obvious loose connection. Though most ICDs are very reliable, there have been several alerts on different devices. Failures of circuitry, lock up of software and other problems are known to occur. Interrogation of the ICD will usually fail if any of these situations are present. If the patient does not have routine clinic evaluations, then the battery may become depleted and the device will become either nonfunctional or will not have sufficient power to charge the capacitors to the required voltage for discharge. Occasionally the detection rate is simply set too high. This occurs most commonly after a new drug such as amiodarone or sotalol has been started, but may also be the result of inappropriate programming. The result of the drug therapy may be a slowing of the ventricular tachycardia rate such that it falls below the programmed detection rate. Significant metabolic or electrolyte abnormalities may affect not only the tachycardia rate, but also the amplitude of the signals resulting in undersensing or failure to detect. As noted previously, the addition of extra detection criteria may delay or prevent the ICD from delivering therapy. Use of these modifiers must be done cautiously. Occasionally the patient will sustain a myocardial infarction that will result in a significant change of the intracardiac electrogram. The new electogram may not be a sufficient signal to sense for the purpose of detection. One might also see asynchronous pacing if the bradycardia backup pacing is turned on. Be aware that a patient in close contact with a magnet might have the device deactivated if this feature is present. We have a patient who carried a stereo speaker (they have big magnets inside) and deactivated his ICD.

Though many patients have ICDs that are capable of providing backup pacing support, frequent use of this feature may result in a significant reduction in device longevity. Thus, patients with ICDs often have a separate pacemaker inserted. This does not usually cause a problem unless the ICD can sense the output pulses of the pacemaker. The worst case scenario for this situation is a patient who develops ventricular fibrillation that is not sensed by the pacemaker. The pacemaker would then continue to deliver pacing pulses into the fibrillating myocardium thinking that asystole was present. If the ICD senses these pacing pulses it will interpret them to be QRS complexes and preferentially detect the pacing rate rather than the rate of the fibrillating heart. Therapy would be indefinitely withheld and the patient would never be rescued. For this reason, special care is exercised during the implant of an ICD in a pacemaker patient or a pacemaker in an ICD patient. Be aware that the ICD can also oversense an atrial pacemaker output with similar results.

CORRECTIVE ACTION
Lead related problems virtually always require a surgical procedure. Most physicians feel that if the lead has failed it should be removed due to its large size and the potential interaction with a new lead. A recently implanted lead that has moved or simply has poor sensing performance may be repositioned if its integrity is without question. A failed ICD or one with a depleted battery must be replaced. Reprogramming of the device will resolve issues due to the rate of the tachycardia or if the ICD is withholding therapy due to additional criteria being applied. Interaction with a permanent pacemaker may be eliminated by programming the output and pulse of the pacemaker to a lower value if this can be done safely. Bipolar pacemakers are virtually mandatory if a separate pacemaker is to be used with an ICD. In addition the pacemaker should be either a dedicated bipolar device or one that has bipolar pacing as the "power on reset" polarity. The latter allows the device to begin pacing in the bipolar mode if its power is temporarily interrupted rather than being reset to the unipolar polarity (see below).

FAILURE TO CONVERT ARRHYTHMIA

The tachycardia may be detected and therapy delivered without conversion to a more stable rhythm. As with failure to deliver therapy, this may be lethal to the patient. Table 16.2 lists many of the problems that result in delivered therapy that

---

Table 16.2. Failure to convert the arrhythmia

High defibrillation threshold
Poor cardiac substrate
Acute myocardial infarction
Metabolic abnormality
Electrolyte abnormality
Drug therapy
Drug proarrhythmia
High voltage lead fracture
High voltage lead insulation failure
High voltage lead migration
Inappropriate device programming
Low shock energy
Ineffective polarity
Suboptimal pulse duration ("tilt")
Ineffective pacing sequence
Pacemaker polarity switch
Atrial arrhythmias

16

fails to restore normal rhythm. Although the ICD may perform properly when implanted, the patient may experience additional changes in substrate that may make rhythm conversion difficult or impossible. If an acute myocardial infarction occurs or a severe electrolyte or metabolic imbalance is present, the heart may not respond to either shock or pacing therapy. Some drugs may increase the defibrillation threshold. Amiodrone is one drug that is very commonly given to patients with life threatening arrhythmias that has the potential to make defibrillation more difficult. Other drugs may be proarrhythmic to the point that the arrhythmia will not convert or resumes immediately after conversion. Fractures or insulation failures related to the lead system will reduce the amount of energy that actually reaches the heart with a marked reduction in efficacy. If a lead has moved it may not be in an optimal position to cause the current to flow through the heart. Programming of the shock energy output to a value below maximum is often done to conserve battery life, allow delivery of therapy more quickly and cause less pain to the patient. However, if an insufficient safety margin is allowed the probability of a successful conversion is reduced. The pulse width of the shock is programmable on some devices and automatic on others. If this is set too short or too long then defibrillation will not be successful. The optimal duration of the pulse is somewhat controversial and will vary based on the resistance of the system. The duration of the positive and negative phase of the shock wave may be programmable as well and can significantly affect the efficiency of the therapy. In some situations anti-tachycardia pacing therapy or a low energy cardioversion meant to convert a relatively stable ventricular tachycardia may accelerate it or lead to ventricular fibrillation. If this occurs the device is usually capable of defibrillating the patient. An anti-tachycardia pacing sequence that is not aggressive enough will not be able to convert ventricular tachycardia either. Finally, it may be that the tachycardia is due to an atrial arrhythmia with a rapidly responding ventricle rather than a primary ventricular arrhythmia. In this situation repeated therapies may be delivered due to a fast ventricular rate caused by an atrial arrhythmia. Though conversion of the atrial arrhythmia may occur from a shock, this is not always the case and the patient may receive multiple shocks. A pacemaker can indirectly cause a failure to convert an arrhythmia. As noted in the previous section on failure to shock, a pacemaker pulse can be interpreted by the pacemaker as a normal QRS. Some pacemakers that have a programmable pacing polarity can have their programming "reset" by the delivery of an external or internal patient shock. The result in the situation of an ICD could cause the pacemaker to change from bipolar to unipolar. If the first shock did not convert the arrhythmia and the pacemaker did not sense the fibrillation, asynchronous pacing would occur. The ICD could sense the unipolar pacing pulses and think that it had terminated the arrhythmia. Unfortunately this would result in the patient continuing to fibrillate with the ICD failing to detect and convert the rhythm.

CORRECTIVE ACTION

If the failure to shock is caused by a reversible metabolic, drug or electrolyte problem these should be corrected. Lead and device issues will likely require a surgical revision. Device programming may be evaluated and corrected if the shock energy is set too low, or if the ATP sequence is not appropriate. Atrial arrhythmias may require drug therapy, ablation therapy aimed at the cause, or ablation of the AV-node. Appropriate pacemaker selection and programming are mandatory. In some cases the pacemaker may require replacement with a new model.

INAPPROPRIATE DELIVERY OF THERAPY

Far more common than failure to convert or failure to deliver therapy, inappropriate shock is present. Often the shock may have been thought by the patient to be inappropriate, but on evaluation of the telemetry data and stored electrograms it is apparent that an arrhythmia was actually present. However, once a determination is made that a shock was not due to an actual ventricular arrhythmia the cause must be found and corrected quickly. Patients do not tolerate repeated shocks as they are quite painful. The patient will often become angry, frustrated and might even demand that the device be removed. Though an inappropriate shock is less likely to result in a patient death than the previous two situations, it must be addressed quickly as in many cases a failure of one or more components is present.

The most common cause of inappropriate shocks is the presence of an atrial arrhythmia and has already been discussed above. Atrial fibrillation is by far the most common arrhythmia leading to spurious shock in our clinic. Many patients who receive ICD implants have enlarged hearts predisposing them to atrial arrhythmias. Another common situation is a patient with a slow ventricular tachycardia who has sinus rates that overlap with the tachycardia rate. Patients who exercise or become emotionally aroused may get their sinus rates into the tachycardia detection zone and receive a shock. Oversensing may also lead to inappropriate detections. Strong electromagnetic interference or myopotentials may cause

---

Table 16.3. Inappropriate delivery of therapy

Oversensing
Electromagnetic interference
Interaction with another implanted device
Lead fracture
Lead insulation failure
Loose connections
Myopotentials
Permanent pacemaker
Detection rate set too low
Supraventricular arrhythmias
Paroxysmal supraventricular tachycardia
Atrial fibrillation
Atrial flutter
Sinus tachycardia

16

detection to occur. We recently published a case of a cable television worker with an ICD who grabbed a live power cable while kneeling in a damp utility tunnel. The AC current passed through his body preventing him from releasing the wire. The ICD sensed the EMI as ventricular fibrillation and shocked the man causing him to be thrown back and release the wire. Most oversensing caused by EMI is not as dramatic as this and is the result of strong electrical fields. A fractured lead or one with failed insulation is a common source of false signals. These leads produce large spurious signals that can be easily sensed by the ICD. If enough of these signals are present and fast enough, detection will occur. As noted in the previous two sections, pacemakers can interact with ICDs. Unipolar pacemakers and some bipolar pacemakers can be easily sensed by the ICD resulting in counting of the QRS, the ventricular pacing pulse, and even the atrial pacing pulse. This would result in the ICD "seeing" a double-sensed ventricular rate of 140 for a VVI paced rate of 70, and a triple-sensed ventricular rate of 210 for a DDD rate of 70.

CORRECTIVE ACTION

The detection rate of the ICD can be increased to avoid overdetecting sinus rates if possible. Occasionally beta blocker therapy may blunt the sinus rates enough to prevent this problem and may be used if tolerated by the patient. Otherwise addition of additional discrimination criteria such as sudden onset or QRS morphology may help if these features are available. The same is true for supraventricular arrhythmias. Ablation therapy of the arrhythmia or the AV-node may be an option in some patients as well. If a device interaction has occurred and reprogramming to a lower output and pulse width and/or bipolar polarity is not possible, a more appropriate pacing system may need to be implanted. In some situations the pacing leads may require repositioning. Lead failures and connection problems will require surgery to correct. The latter should be corrected as soon as possible due to the possibility of failure to defibrillate the patient. If EMI is the cause, patient avoidance of the source is mandatory. For some patients this may involve reassignment of duties at work or even a change of employment.

CONCLUSION

Most ICD malfunctions and pseudomalfunctions are readily diagnosed if the patient history is carefully reviewed, a good X-ray is available, and the data from the device is examined. Unnecessary replacement of the ICD may be avoided and patient safety and comfort may be assured if problems are addressed in this manner by competent personnel.

16

Follow-Up of Implantable Cardioverter Defibrillators

FOLLOW-UP OF IMPLANTABLE CARDIOVERTER DEFIBRILLATORS

Follow-up of patients with an implantable cardioverter defibrillator (ICD) is based on several factors. These patients often have significant underlying cardiac disease requiring regular physician contact. ICDs are similar to pacemakers in that they must be evaluated for capture and sensing thresholds as well as lead integrity. It is not infrequent that asymptomatic ICD lead failure occurs. This would present the possibility of failure to detect an arrhythmia or possibly failure to convert an arrhythmia resulting in obvious consequences. ICD longevity is getting better but many of the implanted devices still have longevity in the 2 to 5 year range. Battery depletion may occur without warning resulting in a device incapable of responding to an arrhythmia. The capacitors of the high voltage circuit must be charged to their full capacity on a periodic basis to maintain their ability to provide therapy.

The rationale for regularly scheduled clinic evaluations is as follows:

1. Allow maximum utilization of the ICD power source without endangering the patient. This is accomplished by programming the bradycardia backup pacing parameters to the lowest output that still provides an adequate safety margin, thus allowing for any periodic changes in capture threshold.
2. Detect ICD system abnormalities through use of the telemetry features and self diagnostic capabilities before symptoms or device failure occur.
3. Permit diagnosis of the nature of device abnormalities before re-operating and allowing correction noninvasively if possible.
4. Allow evaluation and adjustment of therapeutic and detection algorithms, histograms, tachycardia intervals and stored electrograms.
5. Provide an opportunity for continuing patient education regarding their device.
6. Serve as a periodic contact for the patient with the health care system for patients that may otherwise not follow with a physician.
7. Provide updated information concerning patient's location and pacemaker related data should there be a recall or alert for the ICD or lead system.

17

Handbook of Cardiac Pacing, by Charles J. Love. © 1998 Landes Bioscience

A simple ICD clinic is similar to the pacemaker clinic described in chapter 9. In addition to the equipment suggested we strongly recommend that an external defibrillator be available. This may prove useful if an arrhythmia is unintentionally induced during a follow-up session.

PROTOCOL FOR ICD EVALUATION

The methods for evaluating an ICD function will vary depending on the model of device being tested. Pacing function, sensing function and capacitor reformation (charging) is basic to all properly performed checks. The approach to the patient presenting for a routine evaluation at our institution is as follows.

1. Brief patient history related to heart rhythm symptoms, palpitations, shocks, syncope and general cardiovascular status.

2. Examination of the implant site and any additional incisions used for lead, patch or other hardware insertion. Additional directed physical examination such as blood pressure determination, chest and cardiac auscultation are performed as indicated.

3. The patient is attached to an ECG monitor and the baseline cardiac rhythm is observed for proper device function. A recording is made to document proper or aberrant function. Optionally, a 12-lead ECG may also be obtained.

4. The ICD is interrogated and the initial programmed parameters, the measured data and the diagnostic patient data are printed. If arrhythmia detections have occurred and/or therapy has been delivered these data are uploaded to the programmer and printed. These data are evaluated for proper device function and proper response to the patient's needs. Special attention is given to the heart rate intervals and electrograms to assure that these do not appear to be oversensing artifacts. The latter appear as "spikes" rather than a more typical electrogram. Differentiation may be difficult in some situations.

5. While monitored, the patient's intrinsic heart rhythm and, if being paced, the level of pacemaker dependence is determined. This is done by reducing the lower pacing rate of the device to see if an intrinsic (nonpaced) rhythm is present just as is done with a standard pacemaker. The sensing threshold is evaluated by reducing the sensitivity of the ICD until sensing no longer occurs. Many devices use automatic sensing algorithms and do not have adjustable sensitivity. The amplitude of the intrinsic QRS may be determined by direct observation of the telemetered electrogram (Fig. 17.1). The usual method of measurement is from the baseline to the peak of the complex, not from the upper peak to the lower peak. It is important to view the electrograms and to evaluate the quality of the QRS as well as for any evidence of abnormal artifacts that could indicated a lead failure. Most ICDs allow viewing the electrogram generated by the sensing configuration. This is usually from the pacing

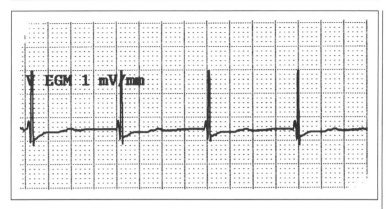

Fig. 17.1. QRS amplitude measurement. This tracing is an intracardiac near field recording. The scale is 1 mV per mm. Using this scale and measuring from the baseline to the peak yields a 12.0 mV signal. This is an excellent signal and will be easily sensed by the device.

tip to the ring electrode. Some are also able to telemeter other configurations such as tip to coil, tip to can and coil to can. These additional configurations allow inspection of the electrogram quality so that any evidence of lead failure may be noted. This may prove very useful in trouble-shooting as the lead impedance of the high voltage system is not easily obtained.

6. The pacing capture threshold is determined by reducing the output until capture is lost. Many devices have semi-automatic methods for determining capture. These enhance the safety and speed of the threshold check in patients who do not have an escape rhythm (pacemaker dependent). This feature should be used routinely due to the safety of this method.

7. Based on the threshold determination, the final pacemaker parameters are programmed. For chronic implants, the voltage is programmed at 1.7 to 2 times the threshold value measured at a pulse width of .3 to .6 msec. Alternatively, if the threshold was measured by keeping the voltage stable and reducing the pulse width, the pulse width may be tripled. The latter method is valid only if the pulse width threshold is .3 msec or less. This does not apply if the patient has anti-tachycardia pacing activated and the bradycardia and tachycardia pacing share the same outputs. Most ICDs now have a separate output setting that is used for the anti-tachycardia pacing as well as for the immediate postshock period when the pacing threshold may be elevated. If the pacing output is shared between the normal, postshock and antitachycardia sections then a larger safety margin will be needed.

8. The patient is provided with a printout of final programming parameters, informing them of the tachycardia detection rate and the backup

17

pacing rate. If the ICD has AV sequential pacing and or sensor-driven pacing ability then they are also told the upper rate.

Adjustments to the device and the frequency of device evaluation should be made with consideration of the level of risk to the individual patient and the requirements of the device manufacturer. Most devices will now automatically reform the capacitors based on an internal clock. If the ICD does not have this feature then the patient must be seen for capacitor reformation as directed by the manufacturer. It is apparent that many ICD lead and epicardial patch models have less than excellent reliability. Because of this it is advisable that a chest X-ray be performed on a regular basis. Whether this is done every 6 months or annually should be based on the lead or patch model and the perceived risk to the patient. We routinely see our patients one month postimplant and then every 6 months thereafter. Repeat testing of the ICD for effectiveness of defibrillation is only done if one or more of the conditions listed in Table 17.1 are present. It should be noted that some physicians perform routine ICD testing one to three months postimplant. Some even perform testing on an annual basis. Additional factors to consider when determining follow-up frequency are listed in Table 17.2.

When an ICD delivers a shock to a patient we ask that the patient call our clinic. The patient is questioned about the events surrounding the shock. If there were symptoms preceding the shock and a single shock corrected the arrhythmia

---

Table 17.1. Reasons for defibrillation testing

Movement of a lead or patch
Questionable defibrillation threshold at implant
Change in drug therapy dose or type
Failure of the ICD to convert an arrhythmia
Failure of the ICD to detect an arrhythmia
Routine testing (as done by some physicians)
Significant change in myocardial substrate
Replacement of the ICD

Table 17.2. Risk considerations for programming and follow-up frequency

Degree of dependency on the pacing section
Device advisories or recalls on the defibrillator, leads or patches
Changes in underlying heart disease
Severity of underlying heart disease
Changes in medication that may affect tachycardia rate
Epicardial patches
Pediatric patients
Exposure to cardioversion, defibrillation or electrocautery
High stimulation thresholds with high programmed outputs
Recurrent shocks
Undersensing, interference or other sensing problems

17

then no further action is usually needed. If multiple shocks are delivered suggesting ineffectiveness of the first shock or a refractory arrhythmia the patient is seen as soon as possible in the clinic. Shocks occurring in a short period of time (but not in sequence for a single arrhythmic event) require that the patient be seen as well. In the latter situation we obtain electrolyte levels and drug levels if indicated. It must be remembered that when an ICD is implanted that there is an expectation that it will be needed. Thus, it is not necessary to see the patient each time it discharges for an apparently appropriate reason in an effective manner.

17

Suggested Reading

1   Barold SS. Modern Cardiac Pacing. Futura Publishing, 1983.

2   Brannon PHB, Johnson R. The internal cardioverter defibrillator: patient-family teaching. Focus on Critical Care 1992; 19(1):41-46.

3   Cooper DK et al. The impact of the automatic implantable cardioverter defibrillator on quality of life. Clin Prog Electrophysiol and Pacing 1986; 4:306.

4   Fabiszewski R, Vollosin KJ. Rate-modulated pacemakers. J Cardiovasc Nursing April 1991; 5:3.

5   Floro J et al. DDI: a new mode for cardiac pacing. Clin Prog Pacing and Electrophysiolgy 1984; 2(3):255.

6   Frye RL. Guidelines for permanent pacemaker implantation. JACC 1984; 4:434.

7   Futterman LG, Lemberg L. Pacemaker update, Part II: atrioventricular synchronous and rate modulated pacemakers. Amer J Critical Care 1993; 2(1):96.

8   Futterman LG, Lemberg L. Pacemaker update Part IV antitachycardia devices. Amer J Critical Care 1993; 2(3):253.

9   Furman S, Hayes D, Holmes D. A Practice of Cardiac Pacing. Futura Publishing, 1993 (3rd edition).

10 Kleinschmidt KM, Stafford MJ. Dual chamber cardiac pacemakers. J Cardiovasc Nursing, April 1991 5:3.

11 Mace RC, Levine P. Pacing Therapy–A Guide To Cardiac Pacing for Optimum Hemodynamic Benefit. Futura Publishing, 1983.

12 Maglione A, Miller J, Reiffel J. Is it sick sinus syndrome? Patient Care Nov, 1986.

13 Mercer ME. The electrophysiology study: a nursing concern. Critical Care Nurse 1987; 7(2):58.

14 Moses HW et al. A Practical Guide to Cardiac Pacing. Little, Brown and Co., 1987.

15 Moser SA, Crawford D Thomas A. Caring for patients with implantable cardioverter defibrillators. Critical Care Nurse 1988; 8(2):52-65.

16 Owen PM. Defibrillating pacemaker patients. Amer J Nursing 1984; 85(9): 1129-1132.

17 Parker MM and Lemberg L. Pacemaker Update 1984, Part IV: DDD Pacemaker-electrocardiographic assessment and problem solving. Heart and Lung 1984; 13(6):687-690.

18 Parker MM and Lemberg, L. Pacemaker update 1984, Part II: the pacemaker syndrome. Heart and Lung 1984; 13(4):448-50.

19 Porterfield L, Porterfield J. What you need to know about today's pacemakers. RN1987; 50(3) 44-49.

20 Sager DP. Current facts on pacemakers and electromagnetic interference. Heart and Lung 1987; 16(2):211-221.

21 Witherell CL. Questions nurses ask about pacemakers. Amer J Nursing 1990; 12: 20-26.

22 Ellenbogen KA, Kay GN, Wikoff BL. Clinical Cardiac Pacing. Philadelphia: W.B. Saunders Co, 1995.

Index